INSIGHTS ON THE "L" WORD

"Bad Sex" by CARROLL STONER
He was rich, handsome, a great date, and "perfect husband material." So what went wrong when the lights went out?

"Crying" by LAURIE ABRAHAM
When you weep and wail in front of a partner, do you get a broad shoulder to cry on? When pigs have wings.

"Pornography" by JANICE ROSENBERG
Do women like to look at pictures of naked men or watch *Debbie Does Dallas*? Janice bets her copy of *Playgirl* they secretly do. . . .

"Mortality" by MAGDA KRANCE
Worrying about a spouse's health is one way a woman often shows her love, but dealing with serious illness shows its depths.

"Losing Control" by JANICE SOMERVILLE
She's gaga over a guy, and for one hot summer, she leaps off the edge, knowing she's going to land hard at the end. . . .

REINVENTING LOVE

CARROLL STONER, who edited this volume, originated the idea for it and for *Reinventing Home*, which is also available in a Plume edition. She has been a writer and editor for over twenty years and won the Penney-Missouri Award as editor of the country's best features section at the *Chicago Sun-Times*. The author of *Weddings for Grownups* and the co-author of *All God's Children*, she lives in Chicago, Illinois.

REINVENTING

LOVE

*Six Women Talk About Love,
Lust, Sex, and Romance*

LAURIE ABRAHAM • LAURA GREEN • MAGDA KRANCE
JANICE ROSENBERG • JANICE SOMERVILLE
AND CARROLL STONER

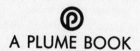

A PLUME BOOK

PLUME
Published by the Penguin Group
Penguin Books USA Inc., 375 Hudson Street,
New York, New York 10014, U.S.A.
Penguin Books Ltd, 27 Wrights Lane, London W8 5TZ, England
Penguin Books Australia Ltd, Ringwood, Victoria, Australia
Penguin Books Canada Ltd, 10 Alcorn Avenue,
Toronto, Ontario, Canada M4V 3B2
Penguin Books (N.Z.) Ltd, 182–190 Wairau Road, Auckland 10, New Zealand

Penguin Books Ltd, Registered Offices:
Harmondsworth, Middlesex, England

First published by Plume, an imprint of New American Library,
a division of Penguin Books USA Inc.

First Printing, June, 1993
10 9 8 7 6 5 4 3 2 1

 REGISTERED TRADEMARK—MARCA REGISTRADA

LIBRARY OF CONGRESS CATALOGING-IN-PUBLICATION DATA

Reinventing love : six women talk about love, lust, sex, and romance /
    Laurie Abraham . . . [et al.].
      p.   cm.
    ISBN 0-452-26991-1
      1. Man-woman relationships—United States.   2. Women—United
States—Sexual behavior.   3. Love—United States.   I. Abraham, Laurie.
HQ801.R343   1993
306.7—dc20   92–38845
                                                          CIP

PRINTED IN THE UNITED STATES OF AMERICA
Set in Janson
Designed by Eve L. Kirch

We dedicate this book to all the men in our lives.

Here's to love!

Carroll Stoner

Magda Krance

Janice Rosenberg

Janice Somerville

We have a lifetime of individuals to thank for helping us develop the confidence it took to write this book. That list starts with our parents and includes husbands, boyfriends, lovers, and men and women friends. More specifically, we want to thank our editor, Alexia Dorszynski, whose intelligence and sensitivity imbue all her work. She and the staff at Penguin/Plume Books, especially Deb Brody, have made writing this book a pleasure. We also want to thank Connie Clausen, whose passion for projects makes her an inspired agent.

CONTENTS

LOVESTRUCK

LETTING GO

COMPLICATIONS

BOUNDARIES

ENDURING LOVE

INTRODUCTION

Why write a book about love, lust, sex, and romance? Could six women writers ranging in age from twenty-eight to fifty and in various stages of married and single lives write about falling in and out of love and what it meant to us? Did we have something to say about coming of age? Could we admit to the uneasy balance of power and authority in the bedroom? Did we want to write about our sex lives and what made them either satisfying or a problem? Could we speak clearly about the conditions that made our male-female relationships worthwhile, and that sometimes made them impossible?

From the beginning, we were committed to this project because we believe that what happens in the ordinary acts of our lives is what defines us. We knew there were many levels of personal discovery we wanted to explore, from our feelings about control and conquest to marital problems and their solutions. This book could not have existed without the meetings that fueled our ideas and our confidence. We swore an oath of confidentiality, as members of women's groups have always done, and yes, some of what we discussed is not included in this book.

In the beginning, the three writers under forty were prepared to be more candid than those of us over that milestone age. When one writer admitted that she had never had such frank discussions, another responded that she talked to her friends about sex all the time. "It comes up when you talk about relationships, doesn't it?" she asked. Well, no, as a matter of fact, for several of us, it hadn't.

Thus, the first conversations were often startling. We were honest, sometimes relentlessly so, whether out of bravado, a sense of competition, or some need to start with our most revealing and frightening confessions and move on from there. In free-range discussions, we told stories about our first sexual experiences and the fear and curiosity that often accompanied them. As if that freed us to speak openly, we went on to describe how we did or did not learn about sex from our mothers and when and where our real learning took place. We discussed the sexual revolution and how it influenced us. We worried about whether we could reconcile work and love. We confided sexual adventures, misjudgments, thrills, damned lies (like faking it, surely the biggest sexual double-edged sword for women), and downright mistakes.

Some themes seemed not to have changed through the years, even in our responses to them. Good girl or bad girl, which did we want to be? Where did we get our ideas about what defined good and bad in terms of sexuality? At home? In the neighborhood? In school or at the movies? At church or temple? Did good mean conventional, while bad meant rebellious and libidinous? And how did self-esteem fit into all of this? We toyed with some strong fantasies, such as being "swept away," and we admitted that many of our worst sexual experiences had occurred when we allowed ourselves to go along with others' demands of us, often after we had drunk too much or somehow kidded ourselves in order to allow our inhibitions to be lowered, against our better judgment if not quite against our will.

Within a few weeks of our first meeting, we began to write. We returned to meetings with essays in draft and completed form. We called them real stories because they are, and we soon realized that some of them were written to figure out unresolved issues, rather than for publication. We analyzed failed first marriages and why several of us had felt so much pressure to be married by a certain age. We talked about the perfect upbringing and how it might have changed everything for us. Several of us discovered, while thinking about this issue, that our mothers had, in fact, made love and sex easier for us.

Within a few months of the start of the project, we had progressed to a point where we could talk about anything at all. Foreplay? Absolutely. Total honesty with the man in your life? Not always smart, we agreed. Sexual fantasies? Of course. Infidelity? Not right, but sometimes tempting. Orgasms? Yes. Out of our shared revelations grew discussions in which sex was only the starting point, the topic that allowed us to open and reveal our beliefs. Why and how we argued, how we resolved conflicts, why some relationships work and others do not, why our first loves were so meaningful and what they revealed—often years later—all grew out of discussions about sex. The point became not what happened when we said yes, but why we said yes or no in the first place.

We were curious about each other, whether we had slept with many men or just one. We know that everyone wants to know about everyone else's sex life and everyone's marriages and whether they work or don't work and why. We tried to decipher why we had behaved as we had. We laughed a lot, sometimes out of embarrassment, more often at the silliness or incongruity of situations and the sheer joy of revealing something and realizing we were not alone. No one ever said, "How could you *do* that? How could you have been so short-sighted?" Our questions were more along the lines of "Why did you do it that way? What inspired that behavior?" Slowly but surely, our writing revealed answers to these and other questions.

The challenge in writing about the commonplace is not in

the attempt to make day-to-day events seem extraordinary, but to tell the truth in such a way that readers find it compelling and meaningful. If a writer succeeds, events become resonant, a version of shared experience. The challenge for the six contributors to *Reinventing Love* was to write honestly about subjects that both fascinate and frighten us—love, lust, sex, and romance—while also making a mindleap over shame, embarrassment, and personal protectiveness. We wrestled with the idea that we might be baring our souls unnecessarily, and that perhaps more of what we discussed should have been left in the confines of a support group. It would be easy to criticize us for going public, for writing about personal subjects that, perhaps, should have been kept private. Still, we persevered, convinced of the importance of what we were writing.

Not that we said everything we wanted to say. We wrote about menstruation, but not in any way we felt was meaningful. We wrote half-essays about abortions (our own and others'), and about our non-sexual friendships with men. But somehow, in the time allotted to writing, we couldn't spell out quite what we wanted to say about these topics. We also worry that this book takes itself a little too seriously, perhaps because we were so concerned about being taken seriously by others. Even in an age of AIDS and rampant sexually transmitted diseases, there is still a lot to laugh about in the subjects of love, lust, sex, and romance.

But perhaps most important, it was validating and deeply encouraging to learn that we could be very different and still understand each other. Talking things over meant we felt affirmed, normal, and far braver than we once had been. We want to pass that on to other women, to tell them that beyond the personal values that inspire behavior there is no right or wrong way to be a sexual woman or man, and that talking about it can be an enlightening process. By the end of a year and a half of writing and talking, our initial feelings of loneliness, embarrassment, and shame had fallen away. In their place was acceptance.

We grew. We changed. Several of us gave up the lasting images of old boyfriends once we had written about them and figured out why they had stayed in our minds for so long. And we put our new thinking to work at home. As one writer put it, "Once I wrote about arguments, we got into fewer fights."

Predictably, there were a few things we never figured out at all, that defied understanding, much less reinvention. Anyone who thinks sex all starts in the mind is unwilling to face what a purely instinctive act it can be. How else can it be transcendent one day and routine another? How can two people wake up at 4 a.m. feeling stressed and worried about the events of yesterday or tomorrow, make love, and fall asleep reassured and feeling better about everything? On the other hand, how can sex on a Friday night with the weekend ahead of you, the lights turned low and the candles ignited, be disappointing? In the long run, we recognize that we are sexual animals with both an instinct for and fear of intimacy. This, of course, is what gives the subjects their nearly magical powers.

And yet love and sex have always been risky for women because our attitudes about them are often a result of our culture's social inequality. Too frequently, we are trapped by our perceptions of how things ought to be, rather than how they really are for us.

We know that women love men and want to like them, too. Most of us want one man to love, and when we marry we work hard to keep the marriage sound. But the amount of change that has taken place in one generation makes male-female relationships difficult. Reinventing ourselves as women has not been easy. But altering the state of male-female relationships is even more difficult because there are others involved. On the one hand, we have more to say to each other than our parents' generations did. On the other hand, we sometimes say it at a shout. Our new agendas have not been easy for men to accept. After all, who would want to give up being catered to?

We know that double standards still exist, and that they are not good for women or men. Crimes against women are too frequent in the United States. The strong streak of puritanism that continues to influence our behavior needs some rethinking. Sexual liberation has changed things for women, but we don't believe it has had such a major influence on men. Sex is still too often accompanied by a leer because we have allowed men to be guardians of our sexuality. As for morality, women always have been its protectors, perhaps because we have had more to lose through the unplanned consequences of unbridled sexuality. Men seem to have an interest in keeping us in the role of morality's guardians, perhaps because this allows them to be free and open about their appetites. But women, too, are sexual creatures.

We know that none of this is intentional. And that's the problem. To be truly intentional about our lives, women need to be honest and straightforward about love and sex and less involved in the self-deception, fear, and shame that are part of an elaborate system intended to maintain the status quo.

In the course of writing this book, we rediscovered what we had always known: When subjects are discussed, they lose their power to cause pain, which is why the process of reinvention is so powerful. One writer explained the process in this way: "The things too painful to look at I had neatly labeled and put away so I didn't have to think about them. But they were always there influencing my behavior. When you take a closed box off the shelf that is labeled 'losing my virginity wasn't so bad,' and you think really honestly about it and try to put it into context in your life, you see things you have been avoiding. Finally, when you have figured it out, the subject loses its power." Another writer said, "Once you can talk about feelings, you're more comfortable having them, and when you know you're not alone you become more confident."

The sources of our strength became clear while we were writing, and the principles we agree on began to look fairly simple: Women have something to teach each other. Simple, intimate truths are important. We are not defined by our sexuality. But without reinventing a few attitudes about love and sex, perhaps we are not defined at all.

One of this book's contributors put it well: "There's a deep undercurrent of feeling that women should *never* let ourselves go. And because love and sex are where we are our most passionate—where we take our biggest risks and where we can be wild and completely ourselves—it's important to know what it's all about."

The message in *Reinventing Love* is this: Today's women must find ways to create love relationships, intimacy, and romantic images that fit our needs, while we also redefine what is deliberate, and what is nourishing. We should feel free to redefine the most intimate moments of our lives, and the attitudes that inspire them. Only then can we eliminate impossible expectations.

—*Carroll Stoner*, August 1992

AWAKENINGS

First Love

LAURA GREEN

I am old enough to believe in signs. I am listening to one on my desk radio now, Copland's *Rodeo*. The music reminds me of the first boy I loved. It was his favorite piece of classical music and he used to play it for me in his room in a house just off our college campus. While students padded down the sidewalk a few yards beyond the drawn blinds of his windows, he danced for me, leaping and swooping to the music in the confines of that tiny room like a heart about to burst.

Early in the course of this book, I agreed to write about first love, and today is my day to do it. I am glad for this radio station and the announcer's choice, which helps me recall the enormous debt of gratitude I feel for my first boyfriend. That was the word we used—"boyfriend"—but it is the wrong word. "First love" is closer to it, although that sounds like something out of a cheap novel. But he was the first and in my tentative way I loved him. I cannot find the right word for what he was, other than transforming.

I left for college two months after my eighteenth birthday with no way of knowing that the next few years would be among the best and worst of my life. I had loathed high school. Now, after four years of being smart, awkward, and different, I found myself among people who loved to listen to the music I loved, who liked the movies I liked, who under-

stood why I wanted to buy folk art, and who didn't think it
was weird that I wore Levis on some days and pleated skirts
and white blouses on others. I had finally moved from the
tight and righteous neighborhood of my childhood into something far more varied and wonderful.

To understand my delight at college, you must also understand that I had almost no dates in high school. From the time
I saw him in my art class, all black eyes and black hair, I had
a hopeless crush on a boy who turned out to be gay. Many
years after I had moved to Chicago, I met him again when I
had a bicycle accident near the steps of the church where he
was choir director. He rushed down the stairs to investigate
the commotion and I recognized him immediately. I had mem-
orized his face. That he was homosexual became apparent as
we talked while he showed me through the church. But when
I was seventeen, all I knew was that I could sit on his lap and
wiggle and twist and lean into him without drawing a response. He sat as still as a rabbit in the underbrush and made
me feel like his predator. Like an idiot, I thought I was the
only girl in school who could actively repel a boy. If only I
had known the reason wasn't me.

That was my sexual background when I arrived at college,
wary and eager. My little circle of friends had all gone off to
liberal arts schools, or moved to Greenwich Village, or stayed
at home. I didn't make close friends in college, but I found a
few I liked enough to make it a roaring good time. I was
delighted to see that young women could be smart in a hundred different ways and use that intelligence for wild reasons
as well as scholarly ones.

In addition to teaching stubborn, smartass kids like me
the rudiments of thinking, college in the sixties was the best
matchmaking device in America. Everything about a college
campus was designed to throw young men and women together. Classes, student centers, libraries, cheap concerts and
cheaper movies, bookstores, coffee shops—if you didn't meet

a man you could love, it was because you didn't want to. By homecoming I had met someone. We found ways to bump into each other at all those kinds of places, more by design than chance. I began dressing very carefully to go to the library after dinner. Soon we were going to the $1 movies at the film guild. Before Christmas break, we had joined the row of couples kissing goodnight outside the dormitory at curfew time.

Curfew was a curious ritual that seems as old-fashioned as a corset, but remember, this was the early sixties, the last dark night before the dawn of the sexual revolution. Colleges wanted to throw us together, but not *that* together. In those years, college administrations did everything in their power to keep the lid on our sexuality. The deans locked us up in dormitories and watched us like sheepdogs guarding their frisky flocks. The school forbade beer, which we drank anyway. As hard as it tried, the university could not keep us from losing our virginity, so it did the next best thing and forced the most passionate and reckless among us to make love in uncomfortable places. Until the ground froze solid as a brick in November, the school arboretum was filled with couples writhing and moaning between two blankets. On one botany-class hike through the woods, our teaching assistant, a naive graduate student who wore her hair in a crown of braids like a Swedish princess, stopped in a clearing to point out something in a tree. As she chattered, the rest of us counted the spent and collapsed condoms at our feet. I heard about someone who got pregnant in the top-floor stacks of the graduate library, where a flock of butterflies lived and few students ever visited. There weren't many cars on campus, but if they had wanted to, their owners could have rented them by the hour.

Boys could stay out at night as long as they wanted but girls had to sign in and out of the dorms after dinner. Head residents watched us leave and checked us in at curfew. We

had to be back in the dorm at 11 p.m. on weeknights and
midnight on Friday and Saturday. Boys could only visit us in
the dorm's tiny living room and everybody had to keep both
feet on the floor at all times. As if we would have done otherwise. Even I, who was dying to break the rules, would sooner
have run naked through the deep Midwestern snows than throw a
leg over a man on those hard little Queen Anne couches in
the Helen Newberry Residence for Ladies. We had our reputations to think of.

Reputations. It sounds quaint now, but I worried about
my reputation. We all did. The system made for terrible hy-
pocrisy. Rather than admit we were sexual creatures with sexual yearnings, most girls drew the line at outright intercourse
and haggled about the cutoff point. It led to the evening ritual
of the goodnight kiss, the closest thing to public fornication
ever seen on a Big Ten campus. Couples lined the walk to the
dormitory front door at 10:50 every night, arms wrapped
about each other. We hugged and squirmed, kissed and
groaned with the pain of unfulfilled lust, swaying like trees in
a storm. It was the worst kind of sexual teasing. I used to
wrap my cold hands around my boyfriend's back, then, as we
got to know one another better, inside his winter coat, then
inside his sport jacket, and finally against as much of his warm
skin as I could touch after he yanked his shirt out of his slacks.
Willing myself to be oblivious to the other couples, I grew to
know every muscle of his back and the muscular contours of
his warm, hairy chest. I kissed his mouth, his eyes, his stub-
bly chin. I felt his hands run along my sides and pull me
against him. Up and down the walk, boys were whispering
please, please and pressing their girlfriends' hands against the
zippers of their pants.

This sort of sex would have been even more embarrassing
if we had been older, but we were young and eager—and
most of us were hypocrites, too. Contorted, public foreplay
was better than no sex at all, and it let girls say in all honesty

that they were virgins. I suppose it was minimally better for the boys, who, at eighteen, could manage an orgasm under almost every possible condition, and probably did, one by one, in that long shivering line. Straightening their jackets, avoiding each other's eyes, buckling their belts, they walked back to their dorms as we wobbled up to bed, our faces bright red with whisker burns, our bras unhooked and riding up over our breasts as we climbed the stairs.

After months of this nonsense, my boyfriend and I took a drastic step for college students in those years. We rented a room from a nice old lady near campus. It cost us $10 a week and was worth every nickel. I don't remember a conversation in which we decided to become lovers and, furthermore, to do so in a proper bed, but we must have said something. All I remember is that one day after classes I found myself climbing three or four flights of dark, narrow stairs to an attic room with a sloping ceiling, a sink, a little window, and, Oh God, a bed.

I must have been frightened; I must have been trembling. I must have been wondering if it would be no good or if I would be ugly to him. It was none of those things. I remember lying naked against him, staring down, because I had never seen a naked man before. I remember that he laughed quietly and kissed me when he saw my quick glance. I remember loving making love, feeling him inside me, and discovering the power that gives a woman. Some of my friends had told me that sex was overrated and embarrassing. They wondered what the fuss was all about. I didn't. I knew.

It was years before I understood how lucky I had been. He was a wonderful lover, with all a young man's energy and enthusiasm. He adored lovemaking and wasn't ashamed of it. He gloried in its rhythms, and embraced its variety. Sex to him was like jazz, an improvisational melody between players alert to each subtle change in the music. He taught me the alternation of slow, deliberate moves with powerful, loose-

limbed lovemaking in which I was no longer sure where I left
off and he began. I learned not to fear sex and my response
to it, to lose myself in it until I gave up my identity, my
borders and margins, to become part of a bigger, shared self.

It transformed me from someone who felt ugly and pitiful
and unloved into someone who felt valued. Later, when he
was old enough to be allowed to live in an apartment, I spent
as much time in it as I could without being caught, which
meant that we were lovers who never spent a night together.
Some days, I would pace his floor, pouring out a long com-
plaint against my family—I was still a teenager, after all. I
told him about my childhood. He told me he wanted to be a
dancer. He talked about his mother and father. I got drunk
for the first time and threw up all over his bathroom. He
cleaned me up and put me to bed. We made love again and
again. He danced to Copland, leaping like a mountain cat
while I watched. We did our homework together, which
brought us as close to domesticity as undergrads could get
then.

Even though we were very careful, I spent two very long
months afraid I was pregnant, weeping with shame at the idea
of having to tell my mother. The gynecologist who told me I
was going to have a baby and ordered me to call my parents
was a cold and judgmental man, the first of several gynecolo-
gists whose professional interest in vaginas and uteruses was
not matched by an empathy for women. He was wrong, so I
never had to make the trip to the abortionist in Pennsylvania,
but I arranged to borrow the money and I would have gone
if it had been necessary.

When the crisis had passed, my best friend's mother, who
had given me all the support I was afraid to ask of my parents,
sent me a letter that still makes me laugh. Inside the envelope
was a postcard, stamped and addressed to her. It read: "I have
( ), have not ( ), made an appointment with a doctor to be
fitted for a diaphragm. Love, Laura." I took her advice and

began the next phase of a lifelong and frustrating relationship with one contraceptive after another. I felt very grown up and responsible with that diaphragm, although from time to time, as I pinched it together, greased and ready to be inserted, it would fly from my nervous fingers and sail across the room and land somewhere with a tiny plop. I would retrieve it from the homework, the laundry, or the dust mice, clean it off, and start over. It kept things from getting too serious.

After a year or so, we stopped seeing each other. I had gotten the world's worst case of mononucleosis, wound up in the hospital for months, and dropped out of school. My father collapsed and died. My life came apart. I enrolled in a commuter college, met my first husband, and married him in my senior year. We had a real apartment, not a room, with real cast-off furniture, and real jobs. I had reluctantly and unwillingly crossed the line into adulthood. I lost contact with my college love before I knew enough to thank him for his enduring, lavish gift.

I would like to do so now. I wish him grace in life, and success, and an abundance of love in all its forms. I cannot underestimate the value of his legacy. That boy on the cusp of his own manhood accepted me. He listened to me, he took me seriously, he stood by me when I was sick and wasted. He told me I was beautiful, something I had been longing to hear. He was generous with his time and giving of himself. He taught me the basic lesson about lovemaking, which was to do it with every muscle and all my heart. He made me feel worthwhile. He saw me safely out of childhood.

He transformed me.

The Old Boyfriend

JANICE ROSENBERG

A few years ago I spent the summer months writing a novel. It was about a married woman named Margo whose memories collide with her everyday life. At least half of the plot revolves around Margo and Lee, her college boyfriend and first sexual partner. His letters to her, hidden in a shoe box on a closet shelf, serve as a kind of memorial to their failed love.

I don't have any boxes of letters in my closet, but when I wrote my novel I did have an old boyfriend in the back of my mind. I'll call him Adam. He was the only guy I ever seriously loved besides my husband. When I consider other men I might have married, his is the face I see. Because I met my husband, Michael, the month I graduated from high school, I never had a chance to play the field. Knowing the self I was then, I doubt I would have done it anyhow. If I hadn't met Michael, I would have found another steady date. That was the kind of girl I was.

So when it's time for thinking of old boyfriends and what might have been—a daydream I think few women can abandon—I turn to Adam. He liked to say that when we first met I was the funniest girl in fifth grade; I'm sure he considered himself the funniest *person* in fifth grade.

In our class picture Adam most closely resembles Ipana toothpaste's Bucky Beaver. With his dark buzz cut, his face and body still round with baby fat, orthodontia just under way, he isn't one of the boys we ten-year-old girls flock around during recess.

Fast forward to ninth grade, when we meet again. Adam is slim. He has a warm smile, shiny dark hair, and a way of widening his eyes and raising both eyebrows high when he thinks I'm not being absolutely honest. He is smart and intellectual, quick-witted and funny, as I fancy myself to be. We are a perfect match. He likes me. I like him back.

Adam and I spend a lot of time together, in person and on the telephone. We have a million things to talk about. We both read constantly and talk about books. We analyze why our friends—in fact, everybody we know in high school—act the way they do. When he gets his driver's license we frequently tour a section of the North Shore suburbs called the "ravines," stopping at Peacock's Ice Cream Parlor in a romantic strip of lakefront labeled "No Man's Land."

Mentally, we become increasingly intimate, discovering every nuance of each other's being. If this were the 1980s, we might go to bed together. But since it is the early sixties and we are good kids, we don't. Instead we have adventures. We ride the "el" to the Oriental Museum at the University of Chicago, take a nighttime boat cruise on Lake Michigan, do crazy things like wander through O'Hare pretending we have airline tickets to Istanbul.

It's 1963. We are seventeen. In the fall of our senior year Adam asks me to go with him to the Homecoming dance. I am both surprised and not surprised. Yes, we are "just friends." On the other hand, people ask me if we're going together. Lately, when they ask, I have begun to wish that I could say "yes." Suddenly I see it as inevitable, the answer to the puzzle of dating that has been right there in front of us all along: We should be going steady.

What I don't take into account is how much has changed since ninth grade. With my sisterly help, Adam has evolved

from an insecure boy who still feels fat on the inside to someone sleek, outgoing, and witty. The previous spring the "popular" group at school courted him. Serving as his campaign
manager, I helped him get elected senior class treasurer. This
fall, instead of hanging out in the morning with a male friend
or two, Adam stands in the midst of the jostling, laughing in-
crowd in a special hallway designated by tradition and unspoken tribal custom as the territory of the sharp kids.

Adam has changed and so has our friendship. By high
school standards, I am in love. Our first date is dreamy and
romantic. The second, your standard movie and snack. I am
doing okay, being cool, hiding my anxiety about what will
happen next, about whether Adam—the same Adam whom I
have talked to on the telephone almost daily for the past three
years!—will call me. As all boys do then (and maybe now,
too), he has the upper hand. He can call me on Tuesday night
and suggest a movie for Saturday or call another girl, can hold
or not hold my hand, meet me at my locker in the morning
or go off to where the sharp kids gather in their hall. I wait.

I hate the waiting. Without being able to articulate it, I
know that I have been downgraded from friend and equal to
girlfriend and inferior. Our relationship has changed. We both
used to make decisions. Now he has taken total control.

As an old friend who knew us both once pointed out,
Adam's self-image had caught up with his self. And, I now
know, at the exact instant when he invited me to Homecoming, my image of him did the same. Romantic feelings for
Adam soon transformed me from his loyal best-female-pal into
a wimpy, whiny, insecure girlfriend. I wanted more than the
possibility of our going out on Saturday night. I wanted an
absolute guarantee. How I envied those girls wearing over-
sized class rings wound with yarn, the girls cuddled into giant
letter sweaters. I stared at necking hallway couples, wanting
us to be like them.

The end was inevitable. Adam wasn't interested in going

steady. Of course I was a drag, but there was more to it than that. Having tested his sex appeal on me, won me, he was ready to move on. Dating was fun, and he wanted to try his luck with other, more popular, less clingy girls.

I did not take it well. For some weeks I begged him for another chance—invited him to a hayride, called him and cried, bumped into him and cried, wrote him notes that he returned with simple negative answers that made me cry again. I couldn't understand why he didn't like me anymore, why he didn't want to be with me forever after all the gentle, loving things he'd said those nights we'd practiced kissing on my front porch.

And from this you make a novel? Well, half a novel. There was more to it than Margo's unresolved feelings for Lee. But that is the aspect of it that absorbed me most deeply.

It's 1987. I'm sitting at my word processor working on the novel. I'm exactly in the middle, trying to figure out how to write an important chapter about the first time Margo and Lee slept together. I've been slaving over it for days, frustrated by the thing's refusal to take shape. And, although getting it right has become an obsession, is making me crazy, I am enjoying myself immensely.

With the supposed disinterest of a novelist, I've given myself permission to wallow in the past. But there is more than the past here. What I'm really wallowing in is what might have been. Although Adam and I never came close to sleeping together—or maybe *because* we never did—writing my novel's romantic scenes is entertaining, satisfying, and—why deny it?—sexy.

The phone rings. I answer. An unfamiliar voice says, "Hi, this is Adam." I am stunned. I have conjured him. It's the only explanation. The conversation is extremely short. He is in town visiting his parents. He asks if I will have lunch with him the next day. I am as surprised as I was twenty-four years earlier when he asked me to Homecoming. As surprised, delighted, and determined to remain cool. As if he always calls me when he is in town visiting, I answer, "Sure."

In fact I have seen him twice since 1968, each time at a high school reunion. In those nearly twenty years I have married Michael, had two children, earned a master's degree, taken and left two jobs, become a writer. I have been happy and miserable, surrounded by friends and deeply lonely, satisfied and itchy with the need to move on. I have loved my husband and struggled with the bonds of marriage. I have adored family life and daydreamed about living alone in an adobe house near the desert. More than once in recent years I have thought of packing my suitcase, but devotion, love, need, and the terror of being on my own—in approximately equal amounts—have kept me home. In other words, I've lived a normal life.

I have looked at other men. Who hasn't? But at times my looking grew into fixation and pulled me away from Michael in ways that hurt him deeply. To make a complicated story into a simple one, there were a few years when he stopped trusting me. When Adam calls in 1987 our marriage is three years past crisis. We are mostly mended. We've spent months talking about everything and have decided that despite our differences, we love each other and want to stay together. But the old hurts linger.

I know that my lunch with Adam will make Michael jealous. Years ago when we first met (remember, I was eighteen), I told him about Adam, how I'd loved him, and how he'd hurt me. How wonderful he was. Smart, good-looking, popular, funny.

I now know I should not have told Michael all that, but I did, and so I have to tell him about this lunch. I do my best to sound offhand. My heart is pounding. Michael doesn't answer right away. I'm tuned in to him like a shortwave receiver. I can feel myself vibrating with the message he's sending. Within seconds I know I won't have lunch with Adam, and I can't stand it. I'm furious.

Michael is watching television and he keeps his eyes on the news. When a commercial begins he tells me that it sounds like a date. It's not a date, I say in a calm, patronizing voice. It's just lunch with an old friend. My wanting to have lunch with Adam is no different from my wanting to have lunch with any old friend, male or female.

The news resumes. The weighted silence stretches. It isn't a date, I prod him. He shrugs. If you want to do it, go ahead, he says, but it will make me unhappy. He means *unhappy*. The house will resonate with his misery. I will spend days reviving him, being both the cause of his pain and its relief. We have been through this before. Frustration churning in my stomach, I consider my options and come to a conclusion. The thought of going through our old style of unhappiness is more terrible than the thought of missing lunch with Adam.

The next day I call him and suggest that his wife join us for lunch. Over the phone I can see his eyebrows rising.

I had lunch with Adam and his wife. He looked the same. The round outline of his high school face flashed on and off beneath the sharp-edged outline of his face at forty-one. His eyes still sparkled when he smiled and he still bit his nails and wore crisply pressed shirts. He was intense, involved with his work as a lawyer, liberal-minded, skeptical, quizzical.

I went home thinking about him. I continued daydreaming as I completed my novel. That fall I wrote its climax. Margo has moved beyond her feelings for Lee. She loves her husband and they live (almost, but not quite) happily ever after. The ending was predictable and, for its writer, barely satisfying.

I continued to think about my friendship with Adam. It's taken me years to put it into perspective. What finally did it was seeing my younger son turn seventeen. One day it dawned on me that Adam was his age. Adam, who had the power to change my life, was as young and innocent as my son. Unbelievable. My son, like Adam, is a senior in high school. Like Adam, he's funny, smart, charming, eager to date girls. I imagine his finding one he likes and having her become neurotically—yes, I admit it—attached to him. I have no trouble imagining his panic.

I don't think about Adam much anymore. Working on my novel, having lunch with him, and doing the thinking that it's taken to write this essay have helped me see him in the proper light. We're two adults with our own lives who once were teenage friends. That was the best part and it is what I now choose to remember.

Thanks, Mom

LAURIE ABRAHAM

Thank you, Mom, for teaching me everything I ever wanted to know about sex, and, once or twice, more than I thought I wanted to hear.

Born in 1940, my mother came of age during the calm before the storm. In the year she married, 1962, the air was still for most young women, and by the time feminism crackled through later in the decade, they were already set in their ways. In the ways of their mothers. My mother belonged to this group, which is why I consider the clear, sunny light she trained on sex so remarkable.

It's not that my mother did not eventually depart from the

course her own mother had followed. She did. If she had not, I would have nothing good to say about what my mother taught me about her sex. Her mother's first and last words on the subject? "Your father was always kind to me." To my teenage mother, those words came to mean that her father had not forced himself on his wife; that made sex an ugly thing that decent women were not supposed to enjoy.

My mother's "personal growth," as it was called back then, was not a direct result of feminism's tempest, though the change in the weather probably cleared the way for her. Returning to college in 1971, the year my younger sister entered kindergarten, she earned a master's degree in guidance and counseling. The psychological bent of that field opened up a new world for her, one in which she began to explore the reasons for her churning stomach. Until I was in my late teens, I did not know that my mother had been plagued by the stomach upset of repressed emotion for the first eight years of my childhood. So determined was she to play the role of the good mother that she never let on. The smiling woman in the short, sky-blue wool dress, sewn from a *Vogue* pattern, the mother in photos, was the only one I knew. Today, I am not completely sure what caused my mother's pain, although it had something to do with the remoteness of her parents, with her vain attempts to imitate her cool mother. In any event, in reacting to her personal cataclysm, she decided she wanted things to be different for her girls. For one thing, she did not want us to feel shame about sex.

My mother's motivations for enrolling me in a class in human sexuality at our suburban Methodist church were a mystery to me. I was thirteen and could not quite imagine that she had had a past, or had struggled through the throes of adolescence. Nor is it accurate to say that my mother simply enrolled me in the class; in fact, she was a member of the church committee that had planned it. They stole the curriculum from the Unitarians.

I've heard that the church has since become more paro-
chial, but in my mother's time its leaders and members did not
shun other Protestant denominations, or even other religions.
Before we young followers were confirmed, as high school
freshmen, we spent Sundays exploring a Russian Orthodox
church (incense, cool!), a Jewish temple (do we have to wear
the little hats?), and a black Baptist church (could they ever
rock!). My open-minded mother and that church were a match
made in heaven.

The class was held in a bland room typical of church base-
ments everywhere: linoleum floor, brown indoor-outdoor car-
peting, a battered piano in the corner. The nondescript
surroundings did not begin to suggest the exotic images that
filled the makeshift blackboard–movie screen once the door
was shut. The slides featured photographs of couples, well,
doing it. Completely naked! And the men were not just doing
the women, so to speak. We sat on the floor in a semicircle
marveling at the various ways in which men and women could
give each other pleasure. The on-screen lovers looked distinctly different from my mother and father. The women had
long, straight, dark hair, parted in the middle, and the men
much the same, with the added dash of droopy mustaches.
When they were dressed, they wore bell-bottoms and leather
vests with fringe. Since it was 1978, these styles were a bit
dated, but they signaled our faddish minds that these adults
were young enough, "cool" enough, to emulate. The accompa-
nying narration promoted commitment, warned of the emotional perils of sexual relationships not based on trust and
caring, and spelled out the consequences of unprotected sex:
unwanted babies and diseases. The slide shows did not, however, create the impression that sex was in any way scary,
abnormal, or evil outside the confines of marriage. ("Most people choose to wait for marriage to have sex," the friendly,
even-toned narrators suggested, and considering how otherwise truthful they were, I'll forgive the overstatement.) In

addition to the audiovisual aids, two church members led discussions on various topics, including masturbation and homosexuality. They often did most of the talking since we were too embarrassed to utter a word, but though we giggled and squirmed, believe me, we listened. Meanwhile, in another room down the hall, my mother taught the parents of my classmates how they might reinforce what we were learning during our Sunday-night sessions.

No doubt practicing what she preached, my mother raised the topic of sex in our house with some regularity. Not in a casual way. She was the adult, my sister and I were the children; she never wavered in that conviction. Mothers who borrowed their daughters' skintight Jordache jeans or smoked pot with the kids did not impress her. My mother's rap, not surprisingly, resembled that of the filmstrip: Sex was best in caring relationships, of a kind that were difficult for teenagers to have, though they may feel as if they love each other very much. We would probably be happier if we waited until we were older to partake, she observed, but whenever we decided to have sex, we should make sure that we used birth control, which we could get at a family planning clinic. She would help us, but if we'd rather she not know, that was fine, too.

Getting us to listen to all this information was not easy. "Mother, please, I'm never going to have sex," my sister or I would whine. Or, "God, I hate when you talk about this stuff. It's soooo embarrassing." But she persisted, stopping when she sensed we'd absorbed all we were willing or able to, but never letting it rest altogether. She left books around the house that she hoped we might peruse. Taking into account teenagers' propensity to avoid anything their parents suggest, she did not say a word to us about *You: The Psychology of Surviving and Enhancing Your Life* and other such nonjudgmental books written for adolescents who were beginning to ponder sex and drugs and so forth. By keeping quiet, she figured she increased the chances that we'd make a beeline for the bookshelf when she left home—which was exactly what happened.

Though she tried to make sex an accessible topic, she did not rush us into anything we were not ready for. "Dave Brown is a fresh guy," I announced upon coming home from a weeklong camping trip with my sixth-grade class. "He tried to kiss me around the campfire."

"He did!" my mother exclaimed, sharing my indignation. "It sounds like you weren't too happy about that."

"It grossed me out."

She never laughed at us, or treated whatever inquiries we did make as anything less than serious matters. My sister walked in on my parents having sex late one night. They didn't notice Shelley quietly standing at the door, or hear her pad over to my room. She crawled into bed with me, worried that Mom was sick. At twelve, I was only two years older than my sister and not sure how to handle this situation, so the next morning I told my mother. A few hours later, I walked into the living room to see the two of them sitting on the piano bench reading a simple, playful book about sex called *Where Did I Come From?* My mother waved me out; this was a quiet time between them, and she did not want me to demand all the attention, as I had a first child's tendency to do.

When I got my period a year later, I enjoyed plenty of attention. My mother cooked my favorite meal, lasagna, and before we began to eat, she announced that I had had my female bar mitzvah that day. I blushed, but she, my father, my sister, and I raised milk glasses in my honor. We all laughed giddily, partly because it was uncomfortable but partly because my mother had succeeded in making my initiation into womanhood something worth celebrating. As an adolescent, I sometimes could have killed her for insisting on such unseemly displays, but now I am touched by her perseverance and, quite truthfully, awed by her wisdom.

For the result of the careful thought and time she devoted to raising me into a sexually satisfied adult is that I am one. I have had my share of doubts about relationships with men; communication with them has never been as easy for me as competition. But sex itself has fit gracefully into my life, a source of both a searing sense of intimacy and a rollicking good time. For the record, and for the benefit of those misguided moralists who believe openness about sex breeds promiscuity, I should say that I have had relatively few sex partners in my life. I also did not have intercourse until after I graduated from high school, partly because I enjoyed the sexual relationship I had with my steady high school boyfriend so much that I didn't see any need for it. We engaged in what goes under the indelicate name of "heavy petting," during which I first learned the wonder of orgasm and, also, how little it may have to do with what is traditionally considered "sex."

Though the thought did not occur to me until recently, enjoying my body but not having intercourse was more or less what my mother thought best for young people. At the same time, she never would have approved of my lustful adventures outright, as in, "Laurie, it's beautiful that your boyfriend's fondling you in his red Mustang," or anything that approached that kind of specific acknowledgment of what went on in the backseat. That was another of her secrets (although it may have been less a strategy than a mother's unavoidable uneasiness at the thought of her daughter's having sex). She made it clear that she didn't expect me to confide nitty-gritty details about my sex life. Some things were private and should stay that way, she said, giving my sister and me explicit permission to preserve the sense of autonomy and personal self-discovery that are so important to adolescents.

That's why I knew how she would react when I called her recently to relate a new trend. Apparently, growing numbers of East Coast parents are letting their teenage children's boyfriends and girlfriends stay the night. Though several of the parents admitted to a newspaper reporter that they felt uncomfortable when their son's date pranced downstairs for breakfast in T-shirt and panties, they thought sex in the family home somehow provided protection from AIDS. As I expected she would, my mother laughed ruefully. We both agreed that sex might become unbearably tedious if Mom and Dad knew and approved. And the only way the tactic might prevent AIDS, we figured, was if parents surprised their young lovers with a condom check every once in a while.

Having It All

JANICE SOMERVILLE

My mother sits on the hill at the country club, watching us swim in the lake below. The clubhouse behind her is white and gleaming, and the lawn is green and even. The familiar sounds of splashing water, bouncing tennis balls, jingling sailboat masts, and laughing children are muted, as if weighted down by the air.

For years, this picture represented married life for my sisters and for me. We didn't know any mothers who worked and we imagined a life spent watching and waiting. My mother worked much harder than that, of course, and she actively pursued her own interests. But still, none of us ever talked about getting married without adding, "But I don't want to sit at Orchard Lake all day."

Above all, we wanted to escape Michigan, which we saw as one giant suburb. I dreamed of moving to a big city and living like Marlo Thomas, or making discoveries on Egyptian archaeological digs that would force everyone to rewrite the history books. And, alternately inspired by *The Diary of Anne Frank* and *Harriet the Spy*, I wanted to become a famous author. But later, after I had embarked on a career and it had turned into a job, and I had tired of my orange cubicle and squabbling coworkers, a nice afternoon at the lake began to look more appealing.

If I became a free-lance writer, I thought, I wouldn't be stuck in an office all day. I didn't want to work fourteen-hour days churning out computer manuals just to get by; I wanted time to read and write and think and dream. The answer slowly became clear. I would get married, and my husband would debase himself with some high-powered, big-money job while I sponged off him. He would buy me a computer and a beautiful study overlooking a lake or perhaps the ocean, in a beautiful home with enormous picture windows. He would fill the refrigerator with expensive cheeses and fresh fruit for my lunches and furnish me with expensive wool sweaters so that I could at least look the part of a writer.

And it would be easy to have children, too. I never had liked the idea of turning them over to strangers, and I didn't think I had the energy or the patience to be a working mother. I wouldn't be a country-club wife on a hill, however; I'd be A Writer—although I might occasionally carry my work to the beach.

I never took this idea of mate-as-patron seriously, or so I believed. After all, I was not some gold digger who chose her job for its monied men. I was writing, as I'd once dreamed of doing, and supporting myself just fine. I interviewed famous people and had even traveled to Africa on assignment.

I was certain, too, that I had the nerve to live the life of a starving artist, if I chose to. *The Razor's Edge* was my favorite book, and I had tremendous disdain for the woman who left Larry Darrell because she couldn't bear the mouse in his Parisian garret. She gave up the most romantic character I had ever read about, not to mention a great trip up the Himalayas, all because she wanted to live in a nice house.

Mainly, I was convinced I didn't take the idea of finding a rich husband seriously because it would mean I was postponing my life for a man, and worse, one who was hypothetical and highly unlikely, given my social circle and my favorite nightspots, which ran to the bar in a down-at-the-heels Thai restaurant. If I really wanted to free-lance, I believed, I would. I was not like the women in recent magazine articles, immobilized while they waited to get married. They postponed traveling overseas, buying homes, and even selecting dishes because it seemed senseless. They would be getting married any day, and then they would begin their lives. I worked with one perpetually single woman who talked endlessly of the free-lancing career she would begin after her honeymoon. Years and at least one canceled engagement later, she is still working at the same despised office job. The story always depressed me, yet I refused to recognize that I might have the same tendencies.

She and I were not the only ones with such dreams. Nearly all of my women friends, no matter how successful or ambitious or politically correct, have told me of similar dreams. They want to launch consulting businesses, knit and sell sweaters, paint pictures, and open restaurants, among other schemes, all funded by their nonexistent husbands.

But none of us believed we would marry just for money. It would simply happen. I'm not sure where I got this idea, given my tendency to write off dates who whip out their Gold Cards with too much relish, admire BMW's, or have M.B.A.s. Concerning this last, my father accuses me of being shallow and judgmental, and I probably am, but I cannot imagine having intimate bedtime chats about the big copier order that got away.

I was forced to confront how attached I had become to my perfect future, without quite realizing it, when my boyfriend and I began to talk about getting married. I began to realize that my posh yet meaningful life probably was not going to materialize, and that I had believed in it all along. In an uncontrollable burst of honesty I confessed to David that I was nervous because I wanted to free-lance some day and he had just opened his own carpentry business. His main priority is not making money, but rather doing good work, enjoying himself, and charging a fair price (which is exactly the kind of thing I was supposed to be doing while he bought us nice things). "I don't know how we'll afford health insurance," I said. "And what if we want children?" *And what about Italian shoes?* I thought.

He looked into my eyes with conviction and said, "We'll just live simply. We don't need a lot."

I nodded *Oh, yes*, thinking that it sounded very romantic, but also thinking, *Damn, there go my new skis.* It's easy to be nonmaterialistic when you're certain the money is going to come rolling in any day.

I recalled my friend Barb, who didn't recognize and conquer her own misgivings about marrying a high school science teacher until her father, a hard-driving attorney, told her to call the wedding off. She would never be happy on his salary, he said. "You'll be struggling all of your life, and you'll be miserable." She decided she wouldn't be miserable at all; in fact, she'd be incredibly happy to marry Rick—and so she did.

I was beginning to adjust to the idea that if I wanted David—which I did—I would have to make some sacrifices or even earn the money myself, when he said, full of excitement for our future, "You can take a year off to write, or whatever you want to do, and then I'll take a year off and design furniture."

I returned his gaze, hoping that I looked thrilled at the prospect of giving up my beautiful oceanside home with its well-stocked refrigerator. Support him? I thought, horrified. But "Of course. That's only fair," I said, more reluctantly than I care to admit.

I had always assumed that when I married or lived with someone we would be far beyond those dividing-up-the-house-work arguments, which always seemed somewhat quaint. Of course my partner would carry his share of the domestic load, I believed. That I would be expected to carry my share of the financial load was something I had never fully anticipated. I had always considered working a right, not a responsibility.

But realizing this was not enough for my boyfriend. He feared I would awaken some distant day, a working woman by necessity—not choice—and leave him. Or worse, resent him. "I wouldn't want you to feel like you're making a sacrifice to marry me," he told me.

I was tremendously insulted. Who did he think I was, Peg Bundy? That I wanted to sit on the couch all day eating bonbons, with my hand outstretched for my allowance? "We're talking about the rest of my life," he said.

I suddenly saw orange cubicles stretching to eternity. And I was terrified of being a working mother. But I knew he was right. The only thing I would really be sacrificing, after all, was the one thing I had never really wanted—dependency.

I admit it, I still think it would be nice to have beachfront property. But as I am unwilling to switch careers to acquire some, and I don't expect the man I marry to do so, either, I will gladly do without. There isn't even a trade-off.

Being Big

Because I'm big, I became an instant sex goddess when I moved to Greece as a nineteen-year-old college student.

It came as a major surprise to me to be routinely ogled, followed, brushed against, and propositioned by complete strangers. It was not something I had expected or particularly wanted. At times, though, it could be flattering and fun, especially since I often got more attention than my classmates, who were all pretty or cute by American standards, but not statuesque like me. It was something that wasn't dealt with in the foreign-exchange program's brochures, and it certainly wasn't what I was used to back home.

Mine isn't the kind of body you'd see in an ad for swimsuits or stockings—never was, never could be. I've never been cute or perky or pretty in the way that smaller women can be, in the way I envied in high school, before I got more or less comfortable with who I am and how I'm packaged, and how powerfully attractive I can be as I am.

No getting around it, though, I'm big—not jumbo or fat, but big, tall, somewhere between statuesque and Rubenesque. My arms are nicely slender, although sleeves are seldom long enough, and I'm forever being advised by clever salespeople to roll them up for that casually sophisticated look. Just once it would be nice not to strain against the cuffs when they're buttoned, when I can even manage to button them. My breasts are substantial enough to be noticed (and once, in a bar, loudly commented upon by Mike Royko) but not overwhelming. I've got a nice distinct waist, and hips that could be less generous.

I do not diet. I love food—high-quality stuff, not junk—and never found chronic self-deprivation good for the soul. I'm healthy and sensible and moderate—a pint of Ben & Jerry's lasts for days, a box of Godivas for weeks. I do not binge. Thanks to my height, I don't appear to weigh as much as I do, but my weight has edged up into those horrifying digits that get hissed when someone else's fatness comes up in conversation. Sometimes I cringe quietly. Other times I smile and say coolly, "Oh, *really*. That's what *I* weigh!" And watch the critics redden and squirm.

It's the legs, though, whose nonconformity annoys. My father had a prosperous, unexercised belly and, unfairly, slender, well-shaped gams with nicely chiseled ankles—all wasted under his business suits, of course. Being European and of a certain generation, he never wore shorts except to swim. Being American and a child of the sixties, I did, and even miniskirts, when I was in high school and they were first in fashion. I probably shouldn't have; my ankle bones have always been barely discernible, and my knees are fleshy as a cherub's. I've got long, thick legs prone to varicose veins and warm-weather swelling, which I inherited from my mother. "*Belle gambe grosse,*" she was told, admiringly, by an Italian sculptor for whom she modeled in her youth—"beautiful big legs." A Greek painter said the rough equivalent to me as we clambered on the rocks edging the wild northern beaches of his country. About ear-high to me, as most Greek men were, he was astounded by the length of my lower limbs, especially from hip to knee, and undaunted by their columnar shape.

Maybe our kind was made to be appreciated by artists, especially non-American ones. Standards of beauty are not universal, after all. At home, big and sometimes gawky as I am, I was more often a guy's buddy than girlfriend. In Greece, I gained about thirty pounds over the course of six months—not surprisingly, considering the oil-laden moussakas and buttery yogurts, the insistence on second and third servings for guests, and the emotional reinforcement I got for being a pumpkin-shaped Cinderella. I was relentlessly eye-balled, pursued, hounded, courted, sweet-talked, seduced, and even fought over. Maybe it was just because I was a single American whose family was reckless enough to let me go abroad unchaperoned.

Coming home, of course, was a big shock. My sex appeal evaporated with the transatlantic time change. I was no longer a sex object—just a pumpkin. I went on the one serious diet of my life, and regained a reasonable figure, although no amount of dieting or exercise could quite undo the genetic blueprint for my legs.

In this country, stately legs generally go unappreciated and uncomplimented at best, specifically and rudely scorned at worst. Usually the insult is subtle; boots are seldom cut wide enough in the calf, among other minor humiliations. The years of low hems have been a blessing, bestowing gracefulness, elegance, and confidence; I will never again succumb to a straight above-the-knee skirt. I still wear shorts, but not the skintight cutoffs of my foolish youth. At least a few clothing manufacturers have finally understood that even solidly built women like to nurse the fantasy of skinny legs, and now make shorts with leg holes so capacious as to make even the fattest thigh feel unchafed and slender.

Only once in this country did I experience a specific exception to the apparent general preference for Barbie-doll legs, and I will forever cherish the moment. About a dozen years ago, I bumped into a fellow free-lancer at the newsmagazine bureau where we sometimes worked. I was wearing a pretty, albeit rather prissy dress, a cotton *milles-fleurs* print on dark blue with lace trim and little pink buttons—not at all my usual loose, Bohemian style. "Nice legs, Krance!" he said, with genuine appreciation. It was just a passing remark, a brush with flirtation between married friends, but it was so unexpected, so unaccustomed, I still blush with pleasure at the memory.

Do such compliments lose their currency for picture-perfect pretty women, who hear them all the time? Do they take expressed adulation (or lust) for granted with a shrug of the shoulders and a roll of the eyes, or do they appreciate it? I wonder. Perhaps it's gratifying to be conventionally pretty, to be desired by men and envied by women, but does a woman really want to be known principally for having great legs, or great tits, or a great ass? No woman I know would want her boyfriend to swooningly say to another woman, as one creep said to a friend of mine, "Can you believe how lucky I am?" while making the universal hand signal for "shapely babe."

On the other hand, no woman I know wants to be known only for her intellectual or emotional or culinary attributes, either. In recent months I've lost a few pounds and changed my hairstyle, and have enjoyed basking in the resulting compliments from women and men alike. It *is* undeniably wonderful to be noticed, to feel the power of one's own attractiveness, especially if it doesn't conform to fashion-magazine standards.

On an occasional browse through the fashion magazines and the tony boutiques, I am amazed and shocked at what women are expected to spend for the accoutrements of attractiveness. Perhaps I'm living in a time warp, but I have a hard time spending more than thirty bucks for a nice pair of shoes, fifty bucks for a pretty dress or jacket. I pay more when I absolutely have to, but most of the time I manage for less. I dress stylishly and flamboyantly, but it's my own style, concocted from sales, discount stores, designer secondhand shops, and hand-me-downs from wealthy friends and relatives.

Last year my husband was sent to St. John in the U.S. Virgin Islands for two weeks to photograph a bunch of very lithe, very young women for a sports magazine's swimsuit issue. "You're *letting* him go?" several incredulous friends demanded. Well, yes. I was thrilled that he got the job, which paid well. My only real pangs of jealousy pertained to the weather there—eighties and sunny—versus here, where it stayed cloudy, rainy, and cold for almost the entire time he was gone. Knowing that the hours would be grueling, that the models would be sequestered between shoots, and that Steve would mostly be positioned so far away from them that walkie-talkies would be used to convey posing instructions . . . heck, there really wasn't much to be jealous about. Sure, he enjoys looking at beautiful nearly naked women as much as the next guy, and being paid to do so was a nice change of pace from his usual stints of taking pictures of guys in suits for the business magazines. But he also knows he's got it good on the home front. He appreciates and loves me as I am. We fit well together, physically and otherwise.

Big, ultimately, is just a description. It can even be a compliment. I've heard enough compliments in my life to have grown reasonably confident of my own attractiveness, fat ankles and all. I've come to realize that I am far more than the sum of my imperfect assets, and that, ultimately, is what counts.

Bad Sex

CARROLL STONER

Who wants to admit to having had bad sex? An occasional not-totally-thrilling episode is one thing. But if it was consensual, and all of my sexual experiences have been, even those when I was guilty of rotten judgment, then why have I had enough bad sex to want to write about it? The answer: Because at one point in my life, I didn't know what bad sex was, and I think it's an important topic for women to consider. If a mutual goal is to live our lives with more intentionality than we are used to, then understanding and, more important, refusing to deceive ourselves about what constitutes bad sex is crucial.

The worst sex I ever had was with Jack.

That's not quite true. What is true is that the worst sex I ever had with someone who loved me and whom I was trying—trying with all my heart—to love back was with Jack.

But then I have to explain why that's so. Why did he love me, if we had a bad sex life? Maybe it was good for him, but then why was it bad for me? In a good relationship, can this ever be the case, that sex is excellent for one partner and awful for the other? Doesn't that defeat the essential underlying premise of sex, that it is mutually enjoyable and an expression of love? Did this difference have to do with technique or chemistry? And most important, why was I trying to love him if we had bad sex?

Actually, the worst sex I ever had, now that I've stopped to think about it, was sex that never really happened, with an airline pilot I once knew but whose name I've forgotten. This guy was cute, single (noteworthy only because many of the pilots I worked with as a flight attendant were on the prowl and nearly all were married), and most important, he had offered to help me move into a new apartment on a Sunday when he'd be in New York. He showed up at my apartment the night before the move. Now what do you think he had in mind?

I was out. He'd brought a bottle of wine and a six-pack of beer, and he was charming enough to get my roommate to invite him in. He sat with her and a friend and they watched television until I arrived home with my date in tow. Then we all sat around and talked and drank and played gin rummy, a game I have always liked in times of boredom and awkwardness.

The evening wore on, with no sign of anyone's leaving. My date was talking to my roommate. I chatted with my roommate's friend. The pilot was talking to everyone. Nothing was happening. So I did what I have done a few times in my life, something that drives my husband crazy: I got up, said goodnight politely (as if this were normal behavior), and went to bed.

In the middle of the night, I woke up with someone in the twin bed with me, and he had his hands, let's just say, in very personal places. I remember feeling cold fury, and yet with my roommate lying a few feet away and sleeping soundly, I didn't want to make a scene. Trying to be polite (this story tells a lot about what I was like in my early twenties), I moved his hands and told him to get out of my bed. Instantly. He would not and so I pushed him away and got out of bed myself, dragging the bedspread with me into the living room, where I proceeded to lie down on the sofa and have a mild anxiety attack.

He soon came out of the bedroom, sat down on the floor

next to me, and began to talk. He said I should stop denying that I found him attractive (I did), that moving someone was no damned fun (he was right), and that at the very least I should give him some simple human warmth.

I listened, though I wanted to throw him out on his ass. Somewhere in the middle of his reasonable proposal, as if we had something to discuss, I had to smother a laughing fit. As angry as I'd been, this was ridiculous. Then came the clincher. I'd never find anyone else to move me on such short notice, he said with an unmistakable note of "gotcha" in his voice.

A night in bed for a move. A trade. This was the negotiation. What I did was to start laughing so hard I couldn't stop. He stared at me, and called me a cold, heartless bitch. I got up, went into the bedroom for my robe, told my roommate what was going on, and then offered to make him some coffee.

He accepted, we drank coffee and talked about the differences between men and women, and I made up a bed on the sofa. In the morning, we proceeded to move from our apartment in the East Fifties to a rent-controlled place on the Upper West Side.

I've never forgotten his words: "You are the coldest girl I've ever met," he said. I think it was the laughter and my assumption that he would still move me that did it.

Which brings me back to Jack.

He was not, as the pilot had been, a casual friend. Jack stood a good chance of being the real thing. We dated for many months, and were getting, as we said in those days, "serious," which meant a mutual admission that there might be a future for us. But other than kisses good-night, some mutual hugging, and a little circumspect necking on the living room sofa, we didn't act on our attraction for many months. Which was fine with me.

The night we finally made love, it was because we both wanted to. He was smart and handsome and what a friend dubbed "ideal husband material." He was falling in love with me, which is a heady experience. I loved that and although I did not feel as if I loved him, I liked him a lot and thought it *might* be love.

Now here is where the story gets complicated. After our first sexual experience, I knew something was wrong. It wasn't fun. It didn't feel all that good. I wasn't very experienced, and to be honest I wasn't sure it was so bad it couldn't be fixed. Maybe, I thought with what I now know was blind, youthful optimism, it wasn't really that bad. Or maybe it was me. Maybe I *was* cold.

So instead of listening to my instincts—the only thing to listen to when it comes to sex—I sort of lay back and thought of England, just as Victorian women were advised to do. Mostly, I did what women did in those days: I wondered what was wrong with me. This guy was in love with me and he had everything I wanted—a wonderful career, and almost as a bonus, gobs of family money (a mutual friend told me), which meant life was easy for him. And therefore for me. So in this case I viewed sex as a kind of trade, albeit a slightly more complicated one than my pilot friend had had in mind.

I had always known I'd marry someone with a certain level of earning power, because I like confident, smart men. Although I dallied with a few working-class and thus dangerous boys in my Midwestern high school (both to drive my mother crazy and to flirt with danger), I knew I would never marry one. Jack was not just well educated and with good prospects, he had a breathtaking amount of money and, even better, knew how to enjoy it. He loved boats and at twenty-six owned one so big it carried a full-sized sailboat as a life-boat. He was good-looking and a product of the best schools in America.

Oh, how I wanted to love this perfect man.

In defense of my behavior, let me explain that I was twenty-two or twenty-three, a small-town Midwestern girl living in New York and meeting my first graduates of schools like Exe-

ter and St. Paul's and Princeton and Yale. So foreign, so exotic, so unmistakably Eastern. Not exactly without resources
of my own, I was tall and slim and with what a boss would
later tell me was officer's bearing (enough years later that he
didn't say officer's *wife's* bearing), and although not beautiful,
attractive enough to catch men's eyes. Having broken the requisite number of male hearts in high school and college, I was
growing confident about my sex appeal. I saw these qualities
as commodities, and yes, I felt expensive. Part of my price
was not being too easily won. Sex, after all, was the highest
card women held in those years—and anyone who tells you
she didn't think that way either wasn't playing the game or
was kidding herself, then or now. The stakes—marriage and
our futures—were high.

There was the undeniable fact that I wanted a life of sophistication, and that some of our evenings bordered on the
decadent: tenth-row theater tickets to the hottest shows on
Broadway, bought at the last minute at scalper's prices. (On
my own, I bought cheap tickets for Lincoln Center or stood
in line for discounted theater seats.) One evening six of us
drank the entire stock of expensive champagne at two or three
bars on the Upper East Side (not the kind, I might point out,
that specialize in champagne), just because we didn't want to
go far. Mostly, we started evenings at the Sherry Netherland's
bar before we moved on to chic restaurants for dinner. And,
of course, there were boating weekends in the summer and
ski weekends in the winter. I liked the life.

It was on his small sailboat, having sailed off from the big
boat to be alone, on one of those perfect summer days when
the sky is almost unbelievably, postcard blue, that I got my
first clue that we had very different attitudes about sex.

Jack was sprawled with his hands hooked behind his head.
Our legs were intertwined. He looked at me with a gleam in
his eye and I was sure I knew what was coming. But no, that
wasn't it. Throwing his arms out, he shouted, "I love being

young and rich and good-looking." We both laughed hard, in love with his audacity, our confidence, our youth. He was in love with me. I was in love with the idea of him.

I manipulated myself into position and started to unbutton his shirt, making my desire clear. What a great place to make love, I think I said, either out loud or in body language. "Here?" he said, astonished. "Where everyone can see us?" I looked around and saw no one other than a few boats so far away that I didn't think they'd be able to make out what we were doing. "Screw out here in the open?" he asked.

I think I gave him a swat and made him laugh. Needless to say, we didn't rock the boat. In my naivete, or whatever it is that makes people unwilling to face reality, I didn't make the connection that when it came to sex we were not even on the same boat.

When we did make love, it was late at night and in the dark. Because I shared an apartment with a roommate, he often checked us into a hotel room, and once, for a special evening, into a beautiful suite. The surroundings may have been grand, but the act of sex was a brief encounter. We were in our early twenties, but there were no nights of passion, no joking about sex or talk of pleasing each other, no uninhibited dancing or fun during or after lovemaking, no feeling of being swept away, and little of the sensuality or raw energy I was just learning to expect. He left satisfied (maybe, although I'm not sure about that), and I did not. I'm not talking about orgasms, although those too were absent for me. I felt responsible for that. In the parlance of the day, I wondered if I might be frigid.

Of course I tried to teach him, but except for one incident, he did not prove an apt student. Once, I climbed into the shower with him, soaped and rubbed his back, and started a little mild sex play. He went from silent, stony embarrassment to liking it. Sort of. But I was too inexperienced to enjoy the role of teacher.

A while later I vacationed in a wild, remote place with the other man in my life, a sweet guy who told me he couldn't live without me and made me believe it. We initiated a sex life, it worked, and in the excitement of things I missed the fact that I didn't love him either. We eloped.

So what is the point of my recollection?

Eventually I had to admit to myself that although his money and power were seductive, Jack was not. And it all came to a bad end, though one that would drag out for months until I told him, after bolstering my courage with vodka, that I hated the way he carried his money, the bills crumpled up in a careless wad, as only someone who felt that casual about money could do, and that I especially hated the way he made love. It all came tumbling out. It was not pretty.

Some years later, after I was divorced from my first husband, I married a man I'd fallen in love with the first night I met him. The chemistry was so great that when we danced and he ran his hand down my back I didn't want his hands ever to stop.

I know now that being with someone who doesn't make your heart beat faster has to be one of the worst things that can happen to a woman. I sometimes think when I meet someone hard and cold that she has never been humbled by her own sexual need or warmed by passion for someone other than herself. Sexless marriages must be awful.

To this day, I cannot explain the presence of physical attraction or the lack of it. To attempt to describe it, I mention the slight movement in the heart, the small skip, or a catch in your breath or a shiver when you think about making love with someone you're crazy about. As for the actual act, whether it is brief or prolonged, there should always be mutual satisfaction and pleasure. When sex and passion are great, of course, it is as close to an out-of-body experience as I hope ever to have. The secret, it seems to me, is having a partner who is intent on giving pleasure as well as taking it. That part must be mutual. To be good, lovemaking must be done with no sense of shame or embarrassment, which I now believe was the source of Jack's problem. (He didn't marry until his thirties, when he met a beautiful brunette. They proceeded to have five children in about six years. I hear it's a wonderful marriage.)

I believe that if you're very, very lucky, at whatever age you marry you will choose the right mate and that sex will be a source of pleasure and comfort all your life. I know that bad sex is far more complicated than the kind that works. I also know that it can never, ever be part of the delicate, unspoken negotiations that precede every marriage.

Satisfaction

JANICE ROSENBERG

The summer I turned eighteen, I read *Sex and the Single Girl* and loved it. I found it fascinating. Exciting. Parts of it definitely turned me on. I admit I looked up a lot of words. One of them was "orgasm." So that's what it was all about. More or less. The book never really said what women were supposed to feel or what specifically you did in bed, but, pun intended, it aroused my already budding interest.

Not that I knew what to do with my newfound knowledge. I certainly wouldn't have used it with Eddie, the last guy I dated in high school. He was two years older, a sophomore in college, and he had a reputation in our crowd for being

fast. It was no secret that he'd been sleeping with his previous
girlfriend.

On our first date, Eddie and I went to a movie. He parked
the car near the theater. I started to get out, but he pulled
me close. As he nuzzled my neck, I remember thinking about
some adolescent graffiti I'd seen for years in the local amusement park's tunnel of love: "Roman hands and Russian fingers." I'd known Eddie for a long time, always wanted him
for a boyfriend, but here I was in the front seat wondering
what to do.

I had figured we might get around to all this eventually,
maybe holding hands in the movie, his arm around me in the
car afterwards, a gentle good-night kiss. In a few more dates
I might be ready to snuggle with him in the car. But this
wasn't snuggling. If I hadn't known him for so long, I might
have been frightened. But this was Eddie, after all, the guy
I'd first seen playing cantor at our synagogue youth group
Friday-night services, the guy who'd given me rides home and
called me on the phone to read me his poetry. He wasn't
dangerous. He just liked to neck.

I, on the other hand, had never considered necking an
activity unto itself. I thought you gave a guy the chance to
neck with you once you'd dated for a while. I never for a
single minute had considered that I, too, might want to neck
just for the fun of it. Whatever Eddie was feeling, I didn't get
it.

After three dates I still didn't get it. Or, closer to the
truth, I didn't allow myself to get it. Why did he want to
grind himself against me and hold me so tight when our relationship was obviously not going to go anywhere? As it turned
out, after all those years of waiting for him, I didn't like him
all that much. He made me nervous. He asked me questions
I couldn't answer. Mainly, though, his blatant sexuality horrified me. After our third date, we had a long talk. I wanted
to tell him that I wasn't ready for his sexy come-on. Instead

I stammered and stuttered about how things just weren't working out. He saved me by saying he thought he was too old for me.

Looking back, I'm not surprised that my long-awaited relationship with Eddie ended after the third date. Through most of high school, I never dated anyone more than three times. It took me years to understand why. The answer, when it finally came, was obvious. The third date was when the real necking started, and necking was an activity I couldn't handle.

How did this prudery come about? Why was I so frightened by the very first steps of sexual activity? When I was growing up my mother told me repeatedly to be careful with boys. "They want to put their hands up your skirt," she said mysteriously, never hinting that I might want to put my own hands there, too. Boys want to get you drunk so that you lose control, I heard, never once thinking that a girl might *want* to lose control.

Her message about sex was as clear as it was one-sided. Boys wanted it. Girls didn't give it away. Any girl who did would lose the boy's respect. The trick was to give it out a little bit at a time, and make boys wait till marriage for the real stuff. What my mother had to say was not about pleasure. It was about manipulation.

How could I move along the path of dating, with its progressive steps toward intimacy, when it would mean going against my mother's insistent warnings? Sex sounded scary and on my own I jumped directly to the conclusion that a girl who enjoyed it must be bad.

Call me dense, but in high school I never figured out that my subconscious could work in diametric opposition to my conscious desires. I wanted a steady boyfriend more than anything in the world. I never dated a boy more than three times. I didn't want to be frightened of sex. I couldn't allow myself the prospect of pleasure. Because these were the only alterna-

tives, I found reasons to dislike boys who liked me. There
was one boy I saw a lot of because he was very tame. I could
control him, and therefore I wasn't afraid. There was another
whom I liked, but he rejected me. Anyone else who called for
a fourth date got the brush-off. My rationalizations varied. He
was too tall. He had a flat nose. He laughed too easily at my
jokes. He wasn't smart enough.

Looking back, I know that every single one of them would
have made a good boyfriend. Because I know that to a one,
they were intelligent, humorous, and interested in me, I am
appalled to think how I treated them. I remember asking one
fourth-date caller to repeat everything he had just said. "I
wasn't paying attention," I said. "I was doing my homework."
The irony is that despite my mother's warnings, she would
have loved for me to have a successful social life, a steady
date, a class ring on a gold chain. As long as I did not get
involved in sex.

So during those important four years of high school, when
many boys and girls are learning their own and each other's
physical responses to necking and petting, my natural sexuality continued to struggle against repression. I told myself, as
teenage girls do, that it wasn't sex I wanted, but love. I knew
the myriad emotions that constituted love, or thought I did.
My knowledge of sexual matters was more basic. I liked the
feeling I got from making out and from fantasizing about making out. I knew guys got erections. I knew that intercourse
meant a penis in a vagina. I even knew that my own dampness
when I was kissing a boy I liked had something to do with
doing it.

If I sensed that the sexual tension I often felt needed release, I never explored the possibilities. Another word I looked
up when I read *Sex and the Single Girl* was "masturbation," and
not simply to discover the real name of something I'd been
doing for years.

Why hadn't I? Can I blame it entirely on my mother?

Years later, when she and I both read Nancy Friday's book *My Mother, Myself*, we had our one and only adult conversation about sex. She said cryptically, "I always moved your hand." I knew what she was talking about. I had two little boys by then and I didn't move their hands.

But that was years later. Flashback to the end of high school. I couldn't wait to get away from home and, although I never thought about it consciously, away from my mother's rules about sex and everything else. I was ready. If I had liked Eddie more, if he had been more sensitive, perhaps he would have been the one. Because just a few weeks later, away from home for the first time, I broke every one of my mother's sexual rules.

At first I got involved with sex because the boy I liked, liked it. No, that's not true. I got involved just as my mother warned me I would, by giving in. I didn't know until much later that I was giving in to myself as much as I was giving in to him.

This boy wanted the same thing Eddie did, but he was willing to neck and pet through various carefully delineated stages on the road toward "going all the way." I knew where this kissing would lead, this touching.

And when I think back, I know that what I liked was the danger of it, the sophistication, the romance, the breaking of rules, probably more than the actual physical feelings. Here I was, on my own, about to do the very thing that I had been warned against for so long. I liked this guy. He liked me. He wanted me to go to bed with him. I went.

Four years later, having finished college and having slept with no one else, I married him. I knew a whole lot more about sex by then, but I still didn't know exactly why a woman would want to do it just for fun. I did it for other reasons. Because my husband liked it. Because I liked being held. Because it gave us a chance to be together at a time when he was very busy. Because that was what couples did. Because, eventually, I wanted children.

I read more books. In *Lady Chatterley's Lover* I read, "she brought herself off against his thigh." By then I knew that meant she had an orgasm. And I had some idea of what *that* meant. Sometimes I almost had one or I thought I might have had one. But it was like the intercom buzzer in our dorm room back in college. If I only *thought* it might have rung that meant it hadn't.

My husband was (and is) a loving person—warm, affectionate, caring, all those things we want from men. He wanted me to enjoy sex, and, as far as things went, I did. Some nights I would claim I'd had an orgasm just to get it over with. I didn't exactly fake it; you can't fake something you've never felt. Instead, I faked a woman faking it. And the reality is that when it came to sex, most nights I wasn't particularly interested. I want to emphasize that I know if I'd asked for anything more, he would have given it. I didn't ask. I didn't know what to ask for. I didn't feel entitled. Sure, as the years passed, I felt cheated and taken advantage of, because sex, after the original thrill of the unknown, had not panned out for me.

Fast forward to a scene I barely remember. A friend is offering me a book. "You're going to like this," she says. She and I have often passed novels back and forth between us. Strangely, she doesn't say anything about the contents of this book, but I have the impression that what she could say would be personal.

The book is *Shared Intimacies* by Lonnie Barbach. It turns out to be the best sex book I have ever read. It goes beyond Helen Gurley Brown, beyond D. H. Lawrence. This book quotes women talking about their sex lives. It tells exactly what they do to have orgasms. It tells its readers—me—that masturbation is normal. (How could I not have known that?)

It encourages me to pursue it until I have a real orgasm. It reassures me that I am not alone. It convinces me.

I take the book into the bedroom with me. Even though I am home alone, I lock the door. I read the book's testimonials about the benefits of vibrators, the value of lubricating jellies, the uses of cucumbers, the varied pleasures women give themselves after their men roll over. And as I read I touch myself gently, tenderly, patiently, as no one has ever touched me before. Slowly I begin to sense what I've been missing. Then more quickly, rapidly, I stroke myself the way I think that men must do from boyhood—and suddenly there's this huge, lovely explosion.

I lie there amazed. I feel wonderful! It was there all the time, just waiting to be released. If it weren't so wonderful to feel it at last, it would be pathetic; I think I knew that even then. How did my friend know what I needed? Or did she need it, too? I would never ask. Five minutes pass and then my hand, on its own, slides back. Does it feel the same way every time?

For a few weeks after that, like an adolescent boy—and I hope for their sakes, like many an adolescent girl—I spend a lot of time having orgasms. I am secretive about it, but I don't feel guilty. I deserve this, I tell myself with the book's approval.

Two months go by. I don't tell my husband. We've known each other a long time, talked about everything but this. This is too revealing. Telling him would mean admitting so much—that I'd faked it, that I'd been resentful of him, that I didn't need him for my pleasure and in fact did better on my own.

Telling him would mean showing him. Of course he'd want to watch. (As the makers of porn movies know, watching someone else's orgasm is highly erotic.) Although I'd seen him have orgasms for years, I'd never really looked at him. It was part of withholding myself. I'd pretended politely, stayed in control, hadn't revealed my sexual self the way he had. I'd been aloof, one eyebrow raised.

So what made me turn the corner? In short, becoming a writer. From childhood on I had wanted to write. That fall when my friend handed me the Barbach book, I had begun writing and was attending a fiction-writing class. I was bowled over by it, by the chance it gave me to encounter myself on the printed page.

My strongest urge to write had come in high school and with its reawakening, adolescence returned in all its intensity. Long-repressed fantasies emerged, creating an excitement that I described at the time as feeling "absolutely crazed." I needed an outlet for a whole range of feelings and sex was an obvious choice. Sex and adolescence and exploration, after all, go together.

Like a daring adolescent, one night after my husband and I made love, when I thought he was asleep, I gave myself an orgasm. It turned out he was not asleep. What he was, was amazed. I told him about my friend's book, how it had freed me. He felt intensely sorry that he hadn't been able to do it for me. I told him he was not responsible. He had done his best. I had never given him a clue that I wanted more. In fact I had never really known I did. I brushed his apologies aside. Then, too, I must have finally recognized I didn't need anyone to give me sexual pleasure.

Having "found myself"—the creative person kept barely alive those married years on a meager diet of knitting, baking, sewing quilts and homemade dresses—I was empowered. I became a writer. I was sexual! I was alive and separate and ready, like an adolescent leaving home, to be on my own, in a way I never had been at eighteen. Then I'd left one safe place for another. Safe from the world, safe from the need to find out who I was, or rather, to let the self I was explore the world. Did it change our sex life? In a word, yes. More importantly, it almost changed my life in a way I did not intend. Freed by my return to writing, I came close to losing everything. But that's another story.

Orgasm. What is there to say? There's nothing like it. No writer has been able to describe it satisfactorily, only to describe it erotically in a way that sends readers to bed, or the bathroom, or to the living room rocker, to experience it for themselves.

Traveling Companions

JANICE SOMERVILLE

The whistle at the train station in Florence was blowing. Antonio looked sadly at me, his wide brown eyes filling with tears. People shouted and jostled us as they raced to catch the train. His friend yelled to him in Italian, grabbing his arm. From the train's windows, faces watched us, some nostalgic, some hopeful.

I planned to run beside the train as it pulled away, waving, tears streaming from my eyes, until it faded from view and the platform was empty. It would be a great finale.

Antonio touched my face, looked intently into my eyes, and shouted to his friend. Exasperated but amused, the friend patted me on the shoulder and shook his head, then boarded the train. Antonio and I watched it roll away. "I will stay with you," he told me.

"Wait a minute," I said, disappointed that my grand farewell scene was not going to transpire after all. "We just met this afternoon."

Antonio, who spoke little English and understood even less, smiled beatifically. My Italian consisted of adding "o" to the end of every word. I wondered how to convey "Get your own room, buddy."

I had been a little nervous about traveling alone in Italy. Everyone who had ever been there, and many more who had not, assured me that I would constantly be surrounded by packs of leering, grabbing, clutching, hissing men. While I waited to board the night train from Paris to Rome, I was thrilled to spot a car filled with nuns. I rushed over to it, but the conductor told me it was booked. There was room at the end of the train, he said. When I opened the door, a carload of soldiers grinned at me, patting their rifles.

I took this as a bad sign, and for the first week of my trip I rushed past all men. I spent a lot of time examining the pavements and buildings, struggling to avoid eye contact. But this grew tiresome, not to mention inconvenient, and I began to realize that I was harassed far more frequently and with a more sinister tone back home in Chicago. These men are only telling me that I'm beautiful, I thought. And not one of them had even touched me. I decided to be more open, if only so that I didn't have to return home and admit that I had never been pinched.

In Florence one afternoon I rested outside the Duomo, mesmerized by its graceful arcs and soothing pinks and blues. I lifted my face toward the warm June sun and closed my eyes, enjoying the soft breeze that rustled the leaves of the tree I leaned against. "*Bella*, no?" a deep voice said.

I instinctively buried my face in a newspaper, but then remembered my resolve and glanced up. An attractive, smiling man in his early twenties was pointing at the Duomo. What was so ominous about that? "It sure is," I said.

"*Bella*, like you," he said and smiled.

I put the newspaper down.

"Your eyes, they are azure," he said.

This is not so bad, I thought.

"You do like David Bowie?" he said and smiled. "I . . . how. . . ." He muttered in Italian and leafed through an English dictionary. He tossed it down and shrugged. "No English, but I try."

He only wants to practice his English, I assured myself. Less than an hour later, we were rolling around the quiet, finely manicured grass of the Boboli Gardens, kissing and laughing.

That was safe, I thought, because he was going back home to Naples that evening. I wouldn't have to worry about giving him false expectations, or fighting him off on a dark street corner. Antonio stayed, however, and so I learned about pizza Napoli, made with capers and sardines, and the bridge with the best view, and the best galleries at the Uffizi. And, as I discovered, he had friends he intended to stay with in town.

Perhaps I have been lucky in that I've never been threatened by any of the men I've met while traveling. I'd like to think I choose wisely, but that would only give me a false and dangerous sense of security. Alternately, I ignore, accept, or embrace the risk. At times I travel sensibly, talking to men only in public places and never revealing where I am staying. At other times, I have looked for men and found them, reveling in the thrill of being in a strange place with a stranger.

Moreover, before the trivialities of affairs and places can seep in, I have returned home. Paris is still romantic to me because I never had to fight its rush-hour traffic on a dreary Monday morning, and so, because we never had to argue about wet towels on the bed, are my memories of the man I met there. I would still rather live in Paris than just visit, and

I prefer a long-term relationship to a string of affairs, but each
has its enticements.

I'm not certain whether I am drawn to so many men on
the road (many more than at home) because they are more
interesting—or whether the settings just make them seem that
way. I suppose it's more of the latter. Just crossing the city
limit makes my libido jump.

It's been that way since high school, when I began marking
my travels not just by the cities I visited but by the men I
met there.

Dave, who lived in Calgary, was my first. I met him in
Daytona Beach my senior year in high school, after my friend
Sue taught me how to pick up men in bars. Heady with this
new power—all I had to do was catch a man's eye, then look
away, then look back again—I spotted Dave across the room
at Big Daddy's while I drank something from a hurricane glass
with an umbrella in it. We spent the evening driving on the
beach in his green convertible Triumph.

In the years since high school, I met Brian at the Lone
Star in New York, Matt in Scotland at his uncle's hunting
lodge, Ian on a steamship going down the Mississippi to New
Orleans, Darryl on the slopes at Steamboat Springs, and Phil-
lip at the National Museum of Kenya. I've lost touch with all
of them, most after a letter or phone call or two. I'm not
opposed to long-distance affairs, but I've found it's usually
better to keep the memory intact than to taint it with too
much reality.

I ruined what would have been one of my most romantic
out-of-town trysts that way. Dan was a successful graphic
artist, witty and sexy, or so I believed in Jamaica. I wish I
could remember only the swim under the starry night, and
the silky Kahlúas afterwards, but unfortunately he paid me a
visit in Chicago. There, between complaints that other artists
stole his ideas and lectures on why I should move to California

for my health, he popped vitamin C tablets by the shaky handful. They minimized stress, he told me.

On the other hand, I still have Antonio's letter, which I always meant to respond to but never did. I read it when I'm lonely and hear him tell me again, under the tree at the Duomo, that I'm *bella* and have azure eyes.

First Love

CARROLL STONER

I had about ten first loves. While each was in progress, it felt like the one, the only, the unique, the special love of my life. Every love gave me a sense of being chosen, or of doing the choosing, both of which were important while I was developing confidence. First loves, although they often end in pain, are about being confident enough to give yourself pleasure. Mine were also about discovery and rebellion, and sex and sin. I learned about others in the exact proportion to what I was willing to reveal about myself. Although I am talking about minds and hearts, it could probably be stretched to include vaginas and penises.

Years ago I read a study that reported that the older women are when they marry, the more contented they feel. Of course. Independence is a great teacher. So are rejection and the ability to reject. But the temptation to choose security and social approval over exploration and unconventional behavior, which defined rebellion when I was young, has always

been a strong lure for girls. Not knowing what our futures
held was painful. When and where I grew up, good girls
married young. But we are getting perilously close to the
moral of this story.

I started falling in love when I was fourteen. Alan had
long, carefully combed Elvis Presley hair that defied gravity.
I couldn't take my eyes off it. He invited me to a movie. We
held hands. The next week he came over to my house and
taught me to play five-card stud. He was quiet but he practiced being a little macho by teaching me and taking charge
in a way that is natural for boys with limited visions of manhood. My memories are of sitting at my kitchen table—a
wooden table painted coral to match the wallpaper—playing
cards and eating out of our refrigerator, which we could reach
without getting up.

What I had with Alan wasn't really love, but the emotional
intensity was strong. We kissed while sitting close together on
the sectional sofa in the living room. I was his first girlfriend.
He was my first boyfriend. I lived for his telephone calls, to
the point that it infuriated my mother, who thought I was
behaving, as she might have put it to a friend, like a damned
fool. It lasted a few months and I don't remember what caused
us to part. I don't think we had much to say to each other.

Alan became part of a group of boys whose main interest
was cars. Today, there's a word to describe them: motorheads.
Then, we called them hoody boys, but they were just working-
class boys with little motivation to succeed. Not college-
bound, they were an interesting contrast to the clean-cut boys
who were. A few straddled the line between the two groups,
getting good grades and being athletic while running with the
wild bunch, but not many. I was mostly interested in the
boys who took risks, and not just on the basketball court. At
the same time, I was unquestionably a member of the good
girls' group. My mother saw from the start that Alan was not
"the caliber" of boy she wanted me to be with, and although

I don't remember her saying anything specific, she let me know this in no uncertain terms, perhaps by raising her eyebrows or slightly wrinkling her nose. Her expectations were clear. My mother expected me to date clean-cut boys headed for college.

After Alan there was a sweet, upwardly mobile boy in my own grade. He was a class leader and we went to the Sun Drive-In after games and ate mountains of french fries and "Sunburgers," multilevel hamburgers that were a forerunner of the Big Mac. We did this with a carful of classmates, but the boys always paid. I was crazy about this boy, when we were with our friends. He had a wry sense of humor and was bright, but mostly I liked being singled out as his girlfriend. It was important to be one of the chosen. For some unfathomable reason, I couldn't stand kissing him. I think he kissed too softly, too tentatively, but I'm not sure. So our relationship was limited to the basketball season, when our pals were around.

Next was Bruce. My memories of Bruce are of the two of us sitting in his car, parked in a private spot that overlooked the city. We didn't have much to say to each other, although he was quite funny. But Bruce had other attributes. He was an excellent kisser. We used to neck for hours. When we moved beyond that, to what we called "above the waist," I remember thinking this was absolutely thrilling, the best thing that had ever happened to me. Although it never included intercourse, or even "below the waist," this was the best sex I would have for many years and I'm still glad I had the courage to take off my sweater. We were both happy with our partial sex life, and Bruce seldom pressured for more.

I can remember as if it were yesterday being held and stroked and kissed. He should have asked me to go steady, but did not, and when he left me and went back to his former girlfriend Sondra, who was a year older, I thought my heart would break. When I saw his car parked outside her house every afternoon for hours (her mother had a job), I figured they were having sex, which doubled my frustration and grief. I never knew whether or not they did it, although my friend Susan tried to find out from Sondy's friend Patty, who said she didn't know. Girls like us kept such things very quiet. My heart mended, quite quickly in fact, though for a while I didn't find anyone who kissed with that wonderful combination of gentleness and passion. Every girl should have a sensuous boy like Bruce in her life.

At the time of my senior Homecoming, I was wildly infatuated with an older boy, Kenneth, who came home from college to take me to the dance. After the football game and before the dance we went to a parking spot where we drank sloe gin. I got drunk, which was explicitly forbidden for cheerleaders (not to mention what my mother would have done if she'd found out). We then proceeded to the dance, where we moved in an inappropriate, grinding slow-dance way and kissed like mad on the dance floor. We did this more to show off than for the pleasure of it, and it must have caused the young teacher-chaperones to talk, since such things were really not done in those years. Later, I confided to my cousin that I hated Kenneth's too-hard kissing. Thank God she didn't hold it against me, since they've been married for thirty years, and who wants to be told her husband can't kiss? (I'm sure she likes it.)

The notion of not being such a good girl was becoming more alluring. I was developing a taste for rebellious, uncontrollable boys—my way of flirting with danger, separating from my mother, and expressing the negative side of my cheerful, good-girl personality. There was one wild boy after another for a while, boys with long hair who did not intend to go to college and who put their limited earnings from crummy jobs into hot cars. They enraged my mother with their bad manners, thereby delighting me. One of them had a car with multiple hand-rubbed coats of candy-apple-red paint and huge flames on both sides.

And then there was a nice, sweet boy again. Ted and I were crazy about each other and couldn't stop talking. We told each other everything. When we weren't in school or asleep in our own beds, we were together or on the phone with each other, having muted, hand-over-the-receiver conversations to block everyone else out and keep from being overheard. Since he was polite and respectable, my mother approved—although my father could not understand, for the life of him, what we had to say during those interminable conversations. But while I was going steady with Ted, my parents bought a telephone with a long cord so that I could drag it around the corner from our family room into the living room and sprawl on the floor in front of the hi-fi set to talk and listen to music. This was back when most families had one telephone, two at the most. I now believe they were cool parents who knew more about what was going on in my head than they let on. After my mother's death a few years later, her best friend told me that my mother had been terribly worried I'd marry young. As she watched my friends marry at eighteen and nineteen and twenty, my mother did not censor her disapproval. Way too young, she said. Get a life of your own first and then marry.

My mother's criticism of my friends made me angry. But I know now that I heard her. Ted was tempting, the first boy with whom I entertained fantasies of marriage, envisioning it as a kind of best-friends, soul-mate partnership. There was only one thing Ted and I couldn't talk about. Since I'd learned a little about carnal pleasures I was no longer content to just neck, and he, from another town and in his first year of college, was an unfortunate half-step behind me in matters of sexuality. Since girls weren't supposed to have more experience than boys, and since he was either afraid or not as adventurous as I, I grew frustrated with just kissing and finally gave

him back his class ring and told him I never wanted to see
him again. He called and called, and I enlisted my mother's
help in avoiding him. I never told him why I had ended it,
or even hinted that it might have something to do with sex
and my desire for him to take the lead. Boys were supposed
to be the aggressors and that was one rule I was not about to
break. Still, I had learned something. With Ted I had my
first meeting of the minds, which I later realized was not to
be taken lightly.

My next love, Charlie, was witty and erudite, good-looking,
somewhat calculating . . . and a snob. I was now a freshmen
in college; he was in medical school. We were both students
at the University of Minnesota, and as Lolly, a mutual friend
explained, it was his insecurity that made Charlie behave like
a jerk.

I gave my first dinner party for this charismatic young
man. I made beef stroganoff (with canned mushrooms) and
my mother allowed me to serve wine, even though I was
under twenty-one and she was a strict teetotaler. I don't think
he was impressed, even though I set the dining room table
with my mother's best china and silver. I'd held about ten
different kinds of jobs by that time and was working at several
during the school year. That night, he was downright disdainful about one of my jobs, which was as a waitress. He
told us that he would never let *his* daughter work. I felt humili-
ated. Soon after this, he broke up with me, saying he wanted
to marry a rich girl, someone from a more polished
background.

In the meantime, I had gotten back at him for his snobbery
by never sleeping with him. I told him that although I was
not a virgin (I was), I wouldn't sleep with him because I knew
he didn't care about me. He protested and explained, many
times, that he was a very good lover, since he'd gone steady
with a girl all through high school and "knew how to please
a woman." I was tempted but never gave in.

I can still remember his smooth, somewhat nasal voice. He was the first sophisticated boy I had ever known. We had dinner dates. We used his parents' season tickets to concerts, and we studied together. My sister recently told me she heard him being paged at the hospital where she works, so I know he made it through medical school. Although I have not thought about him for years, writing this makes me realize I'm still angry. The wounds of early rejections can be very deep.

Soon after he broke up with me, I was approaching a sexual milestone. A tall, confident, and languid boy of twenty-one had moved into his older sister's house on my block. Having laid eyes on him about twice, I developed a crush. When my parents went away on vacation and left me with the house to myself, I invited him over for lunch—a very forward thing to do. We ate grilled-cheese sandwiches and Campbell's tomato soup in my backyard on a blanket nestled among my mother's flower beds—my idea of a romantic gesture. We drank wine and when we finished lunch, I let him seduce me. We made love not twice, not three times, but once. We did not spend hours necking and getting to know each other. We did not talk. I remember thinking that intercourse might be greatly overestimated, that maybe I'd just stick to what I already knew.

I never saw him again, except from my peripheral vision when he waved and I ignored him as I drove into our driveway. But the day we made love he told me he didn't think I had the knack for sex. Although I suspected he was wrong— I'd begun having orgasms while necking some years earlier— this hurt. Terribly. I proceeded to cry for an hour and considered calling my best friend, who I knew would be sympathetic and satisfyingly furious. Ultimately, I decided to keep this humiliation to myself. She had married at eighteen and was beyond such kid stuff.

Why him? I know I hated the idea of my virginity being

someone else's prize. It was *my* sexuality, *my* experience. I also disdained the notion, so popular then, that you had to be "swept away," which somehow relieved you of responsibility in the matter. (As in "I didn't mean to, but I was swept away.") I planned it because that's the kind of person I was. Maybe because I grew up in a home with a schizophrenic half-brother whose presence raised the tension level with an inherent promise of chaos, control is a theme that runs through many of my youthful decisions and probably more recent ones than I care to admit.

Then, too, the idea of "giving away" my virginity annoyed me. The very word "virgin" bothered me then, and still does, sounding as if it should be preceded by "vestal" or "blessed," and therefore part of myth or fairy tale, so synthetic, so man-made. Women don't treasure their virginity nearly as much as men treasure women's virginity. Today's women are far more realistic about all of this than we were. In the long run, virginity is much ado about very little. Choosing a stranger seemed safe, secretive, and put me in control. And he was handsome in the dark, moody way that had always attracted me. In any case, I had done the deed. In some way, I was relieved. I could now get on with my life.

There were a few more boys, but no real sex because I was moving toward what I wanted, which was to get an education and move to New York. By the time I accomplished this I was twenty-one, and I felt instantly at home. I proceeded to fall in love not once but twice during my first year there, and I count these two men as the last of my first loves, since I married soon after and the women's movement came along and changed how I felt about everything, especially love and sex. These final first loves sounded the death knell of my innocence, which is what first love is all about.

Michael was in his mid-twenties, an engineer and former major-league baseball player. He was Italian and the most beautiful man I'd ever seen, with dark, curly hair, almost black eyes, and fine, even features. Brooklyn-born and-raised, he was a neighborhood boy who had graduated from a Catholic boy's high school and a Catholic city college, and he was protective of me, in what I've since learned might be typical Italian good-boy fashion. At the time, I assumed he had a great deal more sexual experience than I did, but I now believe I was wrong.

I shared my apartment with two roommates, and since Michael and I didn't plot and plan, we never made it to the bedroom; we couldn't even find the privacy to neck on the living room sofa. We didn't hang around together as boys and girls had back home, something that created all kinds of opportunities for sexual contact. Instead, we had proper dates. He took me to Jones Beach. We went out for dinner. He took me home, where I met his relatives and I fell in love a little more, with his entire laughing, happy, well-fed family.

I remember Michael's chivalrous behavior. At the beach one day, as we were getting into the car, someone made a sexual gesture at me and I gave him the finger. We were in the car by that time and Michael had a fit, enraged at both the man and me. I laughed and teased him about being possessive. Ethnic differences fascinated me then, as they still do. This was a volatile man, completely different from the practical, matter-of-fact, blond and blue-eyed Northern boys of European descent I'd grown up with in the Midwest. I'll never forget his family's Sunday dinners. They included everything ours had, a roast or a chicken, but with a huge platter of some exotic pasta and an antipasto with more meats and cheeses and olives and exotic vegetables than lettuce. I'd never seen so much food, so carefully purchased and prepared. His family not only ate with gusto, but they talked about food both before and after the meal.

Although I was completely ready to launch an affair, Michael was "serious" about me, which meant he was saving sex for our courtship or marriage. As much as I loved his family,

something about its position in the Italian community bothered me. There seemed to be a lot of suppositions about how
we would live our lives. In one way it attracted me, but the
closeness also scared me to death. I wouldn't be marrying just
Michael. I would be marrying his family and his community
and would soon have a bunch of kids, a row house next to
his parents', and membership in the altar society.

And then, on a blind date with a friend, I met someone I
was crazy about from the moment I laid eyes on him. He too
was incredibly good-looking, tall and dark and like nothing
I'd ever seen in Minnesota. He was verbal and cynical and
tough and funny, not at all protective as Michael had been.
Looking back, I know he never cared deeply for me, but I fell
for him so hard that I refused to pay attention to what seemed
like an unnecessary detail. A law student at Columbia University, he was the top-ranked player on the chess team and said
he intended to play life the way he played chess, a novel idea
for me then.

We talked for hours about everything in the world. With
him, I was something of a blank slate because I thought he
knew everything and because I was so willing to let him be
my teacher. He liked the role. I learned that he too had his
ghosts, mainly a sense of shame about coming from a family
who owned appliance stores in bad neighborhoods. ("A dollar
down, a dollar a week, and send a man around to pick up the
dollar," he said once, looking me straight in the eyes, as if
daring me to disapprove.) When he sent my mother a dozen
roses on her fifty-third birthday, she too was hooked. She
would not live to turn fifty-four, and our love affair would be
over by then anyway. I wanted to tell her how wonderful I
thought sex was, but he was shocked at the notion and convinced me not to say a word. I still regret not telling her and
can almost hear her surprised laughter if I'd had the courage
to do it.

He was my first real lover, and because he was sexually

experienced, the learning process went faster. Had those years
of kissing and foreplay and experimentation prepared me for
great, loving sex? I now think I was more prepared than he
was. Although at the time I thought our sex was great, I know
now that he was not a terribly satisfying lover, since he was
incredibly egocentric and far more interested in his own responses than in mine. Still, we spent hours, sometimes entire
days in bed, surrounded by books and newspapers and food,
getting dressed just long enough to walk up to Columbus Avenue to buy deliciously insubstantial snacks, like miniature pies
and canned soup and cookies and cakes from a Puerto Rican
bakery. I made salads to relieve the monotony of the junk and
smuggled envelopes of Good Seasons Italian dressing into his
apartment on West 109th Street. He thought it was the best
salad dressing he'd ever eaten and I told him it was a secret
family recipe; I had almost no power over him, and I took
what I could get. I later beat him in a chess match after getting
him to promise that if I won he'd never nag me to play again.
I had learned to hate losing at chess.

With him I discovered the basis of all the really important
relationships in my life: competition. While we were doing
everything together, we were also pushing each other to our
limits. It was not a peaceful relationship. I sat through law
school classes to be close to him in an era when there was not
one other woman in the room. We read together and argued
passionately about the meanings of things. We made love in
odd places, including Central Park, on the roof of his building,
and in the stairwell of a West Side museum. It was high
adventure, very different from the carefully delineated steps
I'd taken while parking and necking back home. He possessed
the wild, dark, unconventional streak I have always been attracted to, and still have not seen in many successful men.
Every ounce of the good girl in me responded to the bad boy
in him.

He graduated from law school, joined the Peace Corps,

and moved to South America, where he taught law in Bolivia.
I followed. And until the day I die, I will be able to see
him standing by the fence surrounding the airport waving and
smiling before I landed and ran into his arms. His brown hair
had blond streaks from the sun. I left Oblivia, which I called
it in some feeble attempt to humble him, with a beautiful
wooden bowl that would become a favorite possession, and
with an empty heart, as I admitted for the first time that he
did not love me.

For a long time I counted him as my first love. But it had
all started years earlier. He was the result of a lot of thinking
and acting on what I wanted in life. What *did* I want? To be
with a somewhat unconventional, smart, competitive, witty
man who saw life as I did, and who was confident enough
not to be threatened by the strong woman I was becoming.
Without those earlier boys, our relationship couldn't have existed. Without all of those boys and men (well, maybe I'd
rewrite a few experiences), I wouldn't be who I am today.

It's delicious to think about what we learn from our first
loves. I know now that we respond to and need different kinds
of men at different times in our lives. Mostly, though, my
story is about giving myself permission to take small, safe
steps toward being "bad," which was not really bad at all, but
sexual. I have always been overly concerned with being a good
girl, probably because that became my role in my family when
I was very young. But another part of me was defiant and
dying to take charge of my life. Boyfriends were the easiest
outlet for acting out this little drama. My rebellion was really
about finding bad boys to express what I could not. Fortunately, I had left my appetite for wild boys behind by the
time I met and married my second husband.

Today's young women, it seems to me, are not so bound
up in social approval. They are stronger. They stay single
longer and without fear. Our choices were simpler, more limited. I know a handful of women who were married by nine-

teen because it answered the central questions of their lives: When will I be chosen? When will life begin? Can it still be true, as Adrienne Rich wrote, that "the central temptation of the female condition [is] the temptation of romantic love and surrender?"

As for the pleasures of first love, I don't think the inevitability of its ending should ever diminish one's joy at its arrival. Women should fall in love early and often and marry late. When love starts, we should honor its coming. I hope I can remember this with my daughter and never caution her to avoid its pain.

BENCHMARKS

Sex During Pregnancy

MAGDA KRANCE

One thing we never expected while expecting was great sex. Years before my husband and I got around to having a child, an older man I know who was starting his second family with his second wife described her as having perpetual PMS during her pregnancy—crankiness, crying jags, the works. We were luckier. I was perpetually horny.

At first, of course, there were the breasts. They plumped up and became exquisitely sensitive. At the slightest attention the nipples hardened and sent an erotic jolt straight south, more intensely than ever before. Then there was the constant engorgement down where, in time, I wouldn't be able to see around my roundness without a mirror. The combination made me want more sex more often, to which my pleasantly surprised spouse acquiesced quite happily.

The rest of me plumped up, too, eventually and inevitably. Although little fevers of dismay swept over me when I stepped on the scale, or when I could no longer wriggle into a favorite piece of clothing, my sexual ardor did not suffer the expected inversely proportionate drop. Instead, it distinctly increased. When my husband wasn't around, and sometimes even when he was, I found myself showering more often than ever, and, once I'd washed, gasping at the powerfully intense quick-hit multiorgasmic rush that only a pulsating hand-held shower-massage can provide. (It was a great way to pass the time while leaving the conditioner on my hair for the requisite few minutes.)

"Make love as much as you can now," a friend intoned repeatedly, in the weary voice that accompanies the first months of parenthood. I needed no encouragement. Although we didn't quite re-create the frequency frenzy of our first years together, we came close. The diaphragm, obligatory for so long, was gleefully abandoned in its putty-colored case, along with the crumpled tube of vinegary-smelling spermicide. And my swelling belly became a playful challenge rather than an obstacle.

We took two last-chance pre-baby vacations to the Caribbean. At a time when we should have been starting a trust fund, buying a crib, or doing some other sane and responsible things in preparation for parenthood, our trips were honeymoons for the hell of it, delicious indulgences.

The first was in December, to Saint Marten in the Dutch Antilles, with another couple. I was five months pregnant and feeling blossomy, buoyant, and energetic. The weather at home was utterly miserable—just the way you want it when you're gone. Variously alone or with our friends, we hiked and toured and swam and smooched and nibbled and sipped and slathered aromatic oils on each other. I draped myself in batiked sarongs; with my dark hair, I fancied that I looked like one of Gauguin's ripe Pacific beauties—certainly older than his typical pubescent subjects and lovers, but an engaging image, anyway.

The second trip was in late February, to Jamaica. I spent a few days alone, amused at being unaccompanied and so visibly pregnant, before my husband arrived. The pre-pregnant me wanted to rent a car and explore the island. The real me was well into my third trimester; I felt too ripe to move around much and was content to bask on the clothing-optional beach of the secluded cottage resort we'd chosen, west of Ocho Rios.

Imperfect though my body is, by magazine standards, anyway, I've never suffered from modesty of the flesh. When the
opportunity arises, I happily peel off my bikini top, as I did
every day on that little spit of beach. I had brought along two
maternity swimsuits, but scarcely ever wore them. They made
me feel too frumpy, too conventional, too out of character.

Nude-beach devotees tend to be tolerant, laid-back types.
They smiled benevolently at me, offered loaner beach chairs,
and guessed by my contours that I was carrying a boy. (They
were right.)

Swimming naked, or nearly so, feels magnificently sensual.
Swimming in salty seawater imparts a marvelous sense of
weightlessness, far more than does fresh water. The combination liberated me from the unwieldiness of pregnancy, at least
temporarily. Normally, I would be windsurfing, but my condition precluded that. Instead, I grasped the footstrap of the
sailboard my husband was using, and he towed me half a mile
out to sea. I felt as sleek and graceful (and waistless) as a seal,
and as fast. The swim back, on my own, left me wonderfully
cooled and relaxed.

The Jamaican afternoons were either sweltering or sodden
from sudden cloudbursts. We retreated to the shade of our
high-ceilinged one-room hut to shower the salt from our bodies and then to make waves in each other, in turn languidly
and feverishly. There's almost never time for such afternoon
pleasures at home; with my perpetual state of heightened
arousal, it made us feel deliciously decadent, giddy, and drunk
with love.

The baby came, and the sex went—at least for quite a
while. I even lost interest in the shower-massage. Blame evolu-
tion, and hormones raging in reverse. If, as a species, we all
stayed sexually hyperactive and ignored the needs of our helpless newborns, none of us would be here. Thinking about sex
became almost abstract—I used to do that? Feel that? Really?

It was like reminiscing about a trip to a place unlikely to be visited again in the foreseeable future.

My breasts, of course, became plump udders, devoid of sexual sensation, the objects of my son's adoration and my husband's mild revulsion. Sleep, of course, became the rare and longed-for commodity that it is for so many new parents, the object of fantasy even. Given the choice between sex and sleeping, the latter would win in a heartbeat—even though my heart might long for the languorous pleasures of the former. I knew it was only temporary. Even though I could scarcely imagine it, I knew I would feel passion and lust again some-day. And eventually, I did.

The Silent Treatment

JANICE ROSENBERG

When my husband and I were first married, he was the one who got angry and I was the one who tried to make everything okay again. Looking back, I'm reminded of the old joke about the sadist and the masochist. The masochist begs, "Hit me, hit me," and the sadist responds, "No." My husband never hit me and I never wanted him to, but when he was angry I begged for dialogue and his answer was the silent treatment.

When he was hacked off about something I'd said or done (or not said or done), rather than say so, he acted cool until I noticed. I became extremely good at noticing, quivering like a divining rod or a seismograph. Then I spent nervous hours

trying to determine my transgression, followed by hours trying to force my husband to admit that, to use his phrase, he
had a bone to pick. I wanted everything on the table as fast
as possible—laid out, discussed, resolved, and back to normal.
For many years, this was not to be.

My husband had learned about anger from his father.
When his father was angry, he stopped talking. That was all.
Oh, he continued saying things like "Pass the potatoes" or
"I'm out of clean underwear" or "I'll be home late tonight,"
but his voice was cold. He pulled a shield around himself.
He didn't yell, but neither did he listen. He turned off all
emotions.

When my husband was growing up, his father's anger
could pollute the atmosphere of their home in seconds, like
one of those aerosol bombs for killing fleas. When the family
was least expecting it, some small event set him off. He
stopped talking and they had to guess which of them might
have offended him and how. Because, of course, my husband's
father was always the offended party. Once they guessed, he
accepted their apologies. Sometimes the game went on for
months.

You can use this technique only on people who love you,
people who fear the loss of your love. Anyone else will tell
you to go screw yourself. Well, I loved my husband and he
had the technique down pat.

As for my own childhood experiences, as far as I knew,
my parents never held any kind of long, drawn-out anger
extravaganzas. If my father was angry about something, he
told my mother. And because my mother truly believed that
my father was always right, she accepted his criticism and
apologized. And that was that.

If my mother was ever angry about anything my father
had done, she came right out and said so, too. He listened
patiently, then kindly explained to her that what he'd done or
said was for the best. With little fuss, she accepted his expla-

nation, apologized for questioning him, and, I imagine, reminded herself that he was always right. If somewhere
beneath the surface she stewed, I never knew about it. Perhaps, comparing my father's kindness to her own father's ex-
plosive temper, she simply thanked her lucky stars.

I suppose what I learned in my parents' house was that
men got angry and women acquiesced. The problem was, my
husband lacked my father's magnanimity, and somewhere
deep down, I lacked my mother's faith that he was always
right.

And so to my new marital home. When my husband was
angry, we had standoffs. He turned on the silent treatment
and in no time I began my imploring attempts to find out
why. If, in the midst of one of these situations, we were going
out with friends, he acted as charming and friendly with them
as ever. He also treated me politely. If I slipped my hand into
his, he held it, leading me to believe that his anger was over.
But back home he resumed his cold shoulder as if putting on
some old sweater he kept in a drawer. He turned on the television, picked up a magazine, and made himself comfortable for
late-night solitude.

I never developed his sangfroid. I was simply incapable of
enjoying myself if he was angry with me, because when he
was angry I thought he didn't love me, and if he didn't love
me, nobody did, and then what point was there in going on?
I don't want to imply that I was suicidal. Just hysterical.

Our states of siege progressed like pimples, from the first
sensation of a bump, to the redness, the pain, the ugly pustule
that, if you're a certain kind of person—my kind—you can't
leave alone, that you pick at until it explodes. If my husband
could have, he would have left the whole mess seething under
the surface forever. A bump might rear up now and then, but
he would will it into subsiding. He would never allow the
satisfactory expulsion of the material that had caused it in the

first place. The stuff was just too ugly to look at. As was his anger.

He claimed that his anger would end by itself if I would leave him alone. I said if he would talk about his anger he'd feel better. What I really meant was that *I* would feel better.

It takes two to play the game of silent treatment, the silent one and the one who can't stand the silence. I played because in every instance of anger I saw the risk of total loss. The odds were too high for me ever to say, Why don't you just go to hell? I was too needy to survive the hours of chilly domestic weather. I could never hold out. No principle or preference mattered enough to me. It was easier, and considering my mother's part in the marriage I'd most closely observed, more natural to accept my husband's point of view as right.

He played because, as I eventually understood, in some peculiar way he relished my frenzied persistence. It made him feel loved. And being silent allowed him to keep the deep-down reasons for his anger hidden from both of us. On the surface, his anger was always set off by imperfections in me that he couldn't tolerate. Somewhere below the surface, he was trying to make me into his ideal, the perfect wife, trying to have a perfect marriage, maybe because his parents didn't. And I wasn't living up to his expectations.

The scenes between us embarrass me now to the degree that I find it difficult to describe them in any but the shortest terms. I would move closer to him on the couch and he would shrug me off. I would cry noisily in bed in hope that he would take pity on me. I would light candles on our tiny dinner table and serve fancy desserts. He must have known how much his method hurt me, because sometimes after days or hours of silence, he bought me a present, or simply pulled me close and said it was okay, he knew I hadn't really meant to say or do whatever it was I'd said or done. I accepted blame, apologized, and was forgiven. And things were fine until the next time.

As for my own anger, well, to be angry you need self-confidence and I didn't have much. Early in our marriage when I did express my anger—by slamming things around in the kitchen or shouting or refusing to speak in anything but monosyllables—he responded in one of two ways. Sometimes he treated me like a fly buzzing nearby, not even in his ear, just a small pest that could be brushed away. Other times he managed to turn things around so that he ended up angry with me for being angry with him.

So I learned to keep my anger inside. And, as our marriage progressed, plenty of things made me angry. I was angry at not being able to express myself, at having to accept my husband's theoretical rightness, at having my own anger ignored or turned against me. Though I barely knew that what I felt was anger, I became a walking time bomb. Ironically, that made me the winner in the all-time silence game.

Because one day everything changed. It was one of those turning points that no one would believe if it appeared in fiction. When it happened, we were talking about my newly found work as a writer. I looked at him, heard his assessment of my possibilities and thought, He's wrong, he's absolutely wrong. Believe it or not, I had never had that thought before.

In that moment the power in our marriage shifted like the plates along the San Andreas Fault. My husband didn't recognize it right away, but that didn't matter. I had the power as suddenly as an outfielder has a line-drive ball. I sighed with the pleasure of it, stood taller, realized I no longer had to grovel. I could show my anger. In that startling moment—after months of intense and lonely deliberation about what to do with the rest of my life—the truth came into sharp focus: If push came to shove, I could live it without him.

Emboldened by that realization, I started talking freely, and what I talked about was my anger. For a while, I didn't care if my husband talked. His listening was enough. If what I said made him angry, so be it. The game was over. He could keep silent as long as he liked. I was through begging. Sometimes I asked a question. Sometimes he offered his point of view. Gradually he began to counter my long expositions with short bursts of disclosure. Together we began to investigate the real sources of our anger.

For the first time in our married lives we started having actual arguments. We stated our opinions and backed them up. We took sides and defended them. The essential subject of all our arguments was power and how it would be distributed in our marriage.

Arguing is like needlepoint—you can take it with you any old place. We argued during the commercials in our favorite television shows, in the car on the way to pick up friends, while waiting at the veterinarian's office, on walks taken expressly for the purpose so that the kids would not hear.

On long winter evenings we argued in the bedroom, with the door shut, ostensibly to protect the children's delicate feelings. They would have had to be deaf not to notice, even though they had their door closed and their own argument going full blast. At least they couldn't see us. In the bedroom we soon established an arguing stance. Each of us leaned on one corner of my husband's chest of drawers. He kept the surface covered with an accumulation of small items perfect for stacking, stroking, and rearranging during an argument. Afterwards, my hands always smelled of pennies.

During the day, when the kids were at school or out playing, the kitchen made another excellent arguing spot. I got a lot of work done during the quiet times when my husband was mulling over what I'd said and considering an appropriate response. I wiped counters, put away dishes, scraped dirt from around the edge of the sink for God's sake—anything to keep myself patient with his short withdrawals back into silence.

Why did we bother? If I was so powerful why didn't I just leave? If he was so disillusioned about ever having a perfect marriage, why didn't he? Because we still loved each other. We had these two cute kids we didn't want to hurt. We liked being a family, remembered happier times, were not as brave as we pretended.

Eventually we argued our way through our anger. Some conflicts we settled with careful compromise. Some topics we agreed to disagree on. Some subjects simply lost their voltage. Gradually we stopped arguing, stopped drinking cognac late at night to soothe our nerves.

We still argue now and then, but the arguments are circumscribed. And as for our old ways, anger no longer pollutes the atmosphere of our home. We get it out and get it over with and get on with the pleasant parts of life. I wish that we had been wise enough to do that from the beginning.

Parking

CARROLL STONER

My sexual coming of age would have been entirely different if we hadn't had cars. Parking, as we called it, was how I learned my first lessons about passion and sex, in that order. I feel lucky to have grown up in a small-town-turned-suburb of a big Midwestern city where we had easy access to automobiles, which meant privacy.

When a high school friend, a cool and blue-eyed Scandinavian, married an earthier type who had grown up in the South, I assumed he had far more sexual experience than she. Now, after hearing about decades of a fairly loveless (and sexless) marriage, I think his coming of age was part of the problem. She'd been parking for years. He told her he learned everything he knew in his girlfriend's recreation room.

It's not the same.

Technique, not recipes, may be everything in the kitchen, but it is a marriage of passion and technique that matters in the bedroom. I feel sorry for women who never learned about foreplay and about the potential of women's slower-starting passion. I learned from parking. Parking was not about sex as much as it was about everything that led up to it. Here's how it worked: The boys wanted more than we were willing to give, but for us, they slowed themselves down. We'd kiss for hours, then take what now looks like a tiny step toward the full pleasures of sex, but that then felt monumentally grand— then another and another, until slowly but surely the entire experience of the act of sex became clear.

Interested couples have always found ways to learn about sex. There must be a million ways to come of age. One sad alternative is surely the way my friend's widowed grand-mother confides in a near whisper (knowing I am writing about love and sex): She was a good girl who bled on her wedding sheets but never enjoyed sex during the sixty years she was married. "He never spent time kissing or holding me," she says, shaking her head sadly. What she never learned was how to slow him down, and what she had the right to demand.

That kissing, and kissing alone, is worth knowing about is not something I've thought much about, although I always knew, from those years of parking, that it was an interesting end unto itself. Naturally, as we get older and more sexually experienced, we move eagerly and greedily from kissing to pleasure in larger measure. But in the same way that young

children must first master simple skills, kissing is worth some
time and effort. Ranging from teasing and playful to seriously
erotic, kissing seems as basic as learning the alphabet. I'm sure
a couple who love to kiss for fairly extended periods of time
will develop a good sex life. Prolonged kissing, not necking or
petting, was the most important part of defining desire while
we also learned to control our appetites.

Let me explain parking. There were many private spots in
our suburb: next to empty lots, by parks, by golf courses and,
since this was Minnesota, in the woods that surrounded lakes.
But two major public parking lots, one near a golf course and
the other a scenic overlook of downtown Minneapolis, were
known to attract couples from our town. When you drove into
them you often recognized the cars of friends and classmates.
Saying "There's Wally and Amanda; there's Bonnie and Ron"
made you feel connected, in the know. Parking was a very
cool thing to do. At a time in our lives when being popular
was more important than anything else (even being loved),
parking may have been cool because it was a public statement
that you were desired.

Parking had firm protocol. You never, for instance, spoke
to other couples or acted as if you saw them. You turned off
your lights as you glided into your own spot, as far from other
cars as possible. Only a jerk would have honked or made any
sign of recognition or parked right next to someone. You could
have been run out of school for such a gaffe. You were silent.
I do not recall ever hearing laughter or conversation coming
from other cars, although we often parked in the summer with
our car windows wide open.

Those of us who were concerned about our reputations
didn't worry that parking would damage them. An occasional
car full of boys might cruise by and check out whose cars
were there, guessing whom each boy was with. But the fairly
rigid morality that governed us elsewhere was suspended for
parking. To this day, I assume everyone else was doing what

I was doing and am astonished by a friend's admission that she started having intercourse at fourteen. In her boyfriend's father's car! But most friends confide that, yes, they necked and petted when they parked, did a little unbuttoning and unzipping, but mostly clothes-on stuff. Whatever might be going on, you never, ever talked about what other couples might or might not be doing. I know couples who parked when they were on double dates, but I considered that gross. We wanted to learn about sex. But we wanted privacy while we were learning.

One winter night a boyfriend said he was glad we lived in a cold climate so that the car windows steamed up and no one could see what was going on inside. After that we steamed up the car windows fast, sort of as a joke, so that we were completely enclosed in our own private cocoon. I wonder if I've ever felt as loved or as safe as I felt in that seventeen-year-old boy's arms. I don't think we even locked the car doors. There wasn't much to be protected from, other than each other and the occasional police car that cruised by and shone its lights on cars that looked empty. As soon as we saw the lights, we sat up, and as soon as they saw our heads, they drove away. Once they left, of course, we sprawled out again. Although he was over six feet tall and I was five-seven, I don't remember complaining about sharing our space with the steering wheel. We did not climb into the backseat. That would have been "fast."

I never had a curfew. "I trust my girls," my mother said. Still, she wondered why I had to be away from home every night. The idea of doing any of this in our comfortably furnished recreation room, built for us, was totally out of the question. We had blankets and the car's heater, which we carefully monitored because of the frigid weather outside. We had the radio. And we had each other.

I have a young daughter who is flirting with the idea of liking boys after all. I hope I can watch her infatuations with tolerance and pleasure. We live in the city, and I wonder where young couples go for such experience. Things are different now. There are good reasons to avoid casual sex. But the middle to late teens might still be the most important time for girls to learn about love and sex and women's often more prolonged process of passion.

Early marriages can be disastrous for women, who mature sooner than men but need more time to learn to live outside convention. What necking and petting were about was exploring sexuality while we postponed marriage. With the hindsight of age, and with my mother's warning about the difficulties of early marriage still fresh in my mind, I see chastity as far less important than coming into our sexual selves. And I don't know a single woman who had the nerve to park with her boyfriend for hours in high school or college who has any problems with sex.

Arguments

LAURIE ABRAHAM

"How can you say that people in the ghetto should move to the Southwest to work as migrant laborers?" I fume, picking up my glass and newspaper from the table that sits on our second-floor porch, gathering my supplies for a retreat.

"That's where the jobs are," my lover responds much more calmly. He stays in his lawn chair, his copy of *Anna Karenina* temporarily at rest on his lap. "That's not what I'm saying, anyway. Throughout history people have moved where the jobs are."

"So you're saying the welfare state is preventing people from moving where they should," I snarl from behind the screen door, where I have moved for cover.

"That woman just went inside," Mike accuses. "That woman" is a neighbor who, like us, has been spending a mercilessly hot summer Saturday morning on her porch. Our second-floor porches are separated by only twenty feet of air, and Mike is implying that my shrillness has driven her away. That I am too loud, especially in public, is the subtext that often runs through our main arguments.

It is not unusual for the warfare to begin out on the back porch, while we're reading the newspaper. Outraged at one or another injustice against mankind, I typically say something like "Can you believe that families of four on welfare only get three hundred and sixty-nine dollars a month?" I used to expect Mike to mumble assent, share my indignation for a moment, and then move on. Instead, I hear, "Maybe if they didn't get three hundred and sixty-nine dollars they would go get jobs." For the sake of clarity, I've simplified and compressed our dialogue, but this interchange captures the essence of our arguments.

While I have been known to argue my generally liberal viewpoints to the point of tears, Mike remains calmly apolitical, or if anything, conservative. As I engage, my voice rises; Mike sounds much more pleasant and rational but never, ever backs down. Our true beliefs may be much subtler than would seem evident were you to overhear one of our matches (and of course, Mike assures me that a good number of people have had that opportunity), but in the midst of a fight, positions harden like concrete. Once it's dry, there's no chance to scratch out the message you've written and replace it with a more conciliatory one.

What puzzles me most about our arguments is that we so often debate "issues" (for example, the welfare state). Raised by a woman with Freudian tendencies—my mother believes most arguments about toothpaste tubes are really about more fundamental "relationship" questions too sensitive to be directly addressed—I didn't think couples argued about anything except what went on between them. The relationship, or its shortfalls, fuel the fires. I keep looking for the "real cause" of our arguments, but perhaps the cause is simply our different political views. This notion has been a revelation for me. I remember being surprised to hear friends say that they could not marry Republicans. (I do not have any friends who could not marry a Democrat. Indeed, I wonder: Are there any such women out there?) As a reporter, I've chosen to devote my career to writing about race and poverty issues, and I was deluding myself into thinking that politics would not matter in my personal relationships. And at some level I knew they did, as I've never looked twice at the dark-suited men, the M.B.A. masses.

Until Mike, I had not confronted opposing political leanings in a relationship. In my other relationship, I was the political adviser. If my boyfriend and I couldn't agree on aesthetics—and we couldn't—one thing we could always agree on was that the government was shirking its responsibility to the poor. I thought Mike was more like me when we first got together. He had a master's degree in public policy, a discipline that tends to attract people who believe in a large, activist government because without the government they would be unemployed; he was headed to Yale University to study law (almost all of my attorney acquaintances work for the Legal Aid Society); and he wore small, round, wire-framed glasses. As I came to know him, however, I learned that he was exploring classical liberal ideas, which often boil down to the contention that the government that governs best, governs least.

In the beginning, of course, his politics were about the furthest thing from my mind. I couldn't help blurting out my political views, but I backed off afterward, or argued halfheartedly, maybe even playfully. I liked him; I didn't want to scare him away. (My mother had warned me about being too intense early on in a relationship.) I was blinded by love, or infatuation, or whatever you call that starry-eyed state that is the first stage of romance: the stomach that tightens each time the phone rings; the rediscovery of the siren call of blaring rock and roll; the loopy lists of sights that remind me of *him*— street signs, Mexican grocery stores, Hondas, smokestacks, anything and everything. During that time, my tingling heart and buzzing mind were not capable of receiving any signals that would have detracted from the wonder of him. I do remember, however, that during our second or third date I challenged him about his repeated use of the word "pleasant," a listless, effete word that did not fit into my more passionate, black-and-white view of the world. "Pleasant" sounded so proper, so restrained and noncommittal. I don't remember how Mike responded to my "pleasant"-bashing. He probably thought, "Gee, this is one prickly woman." I couldn't blame him because my feeling about that word seems silly and churlish from a distance, but I think my reaction was telling. Our divergent attitudes toward "pleasant" foreshadowed much of what was to come, which has sometimes been distinctly *un*-pleasant. At the time, of course, I dismissed the warning.

But it was more than a love-high that kept me from discerning Mike's political stripes. He frequently says he doesn't have any. He tells me that his interest in classical liberalism can be separated from politics. He says he's confused; that he is still searching for his political beliefs, that he may never have any. He may not even want them, I've heard him say. Because they would interfere with his intellectual freedom, I suppose. He relishes the stimulation of being contrary. What I haven't yet mentioned is that Mike also holds a doctorate in philosophy, a discipline predicated on the open-ended (I'd say unending) discussion of all points of view. Mike is not compelled to choose one side or the other. Indeed his compulsion runs to *not* taking a position, whereas I consider taking one imperative for responsible living. I've seen Mike argue the liberal side—my side—with other people, but with me, he invariably ends up sounding conservative. Perhaps it would bore him if we agreed, or seem intellectually dishonest, so he leaves all political options open, for the mind-stretching sport of it all.

Be that as it may, in our relationship we both got more than we bargained for. My theory is that Mike at first appreciated my willingness to engage in intellectual sparring, but he has not been pleased with how seriously I take it. To invert an old phrase, the political is personal to me. I take my politics personally and passionately, while Mike keeps his at arm's length.

To give my Freudian mother her due, the vehemence of our arguments cannot be explained away solely by my political zeal. I have an uncommonly strong need to win, to be right, whatever the subject, and especially with men. I still can't help feeling a spark of pride when I remember beating Dave Brown one-on-one in basketball in fifth grade. Perhaps I learned to connect with men by competing with them because my relationship with my father was based on that. We got close on the basketball court and the softball field. To gain respect and a place with men, I strive to be faster, stronger, smarter. I want to beat them at their own games. As a child, maybe Mike was somehow programmed to be a provocateur; maybe he feeds on the energy that flows when we do battle. I don't know. What I do know is that Mike jabs, and I respond: always, always, always.

But the constant skirmishing is wearing us down. We both yearn to agree, to find some common ground. Several times we have discussed *not* discussing issues that cause contention, but we are wary of a relationship that requires such vigilance, in which we must tiptoe around a minefield of taboo subjects. It probably would help if we could step back from our argu-

ments before they get too heated and see if they're worth the
words. But so far, we haven't done that. As is perhaps not
surprising, I'm trying to bring Mike over to my side. I keep
trying to get him to read a book that takes a moderate approach to welfare-state problems, that outlines what I believe
in a thoughtful analysis of the problems and offers some creative, cogent solutions. He says he wants to read it but has
not had the chance with all the academic reading he must
attend to. I doubt he really wants to read such serious stuff
in his free time, though he insists he does. I'm thinking of
bringing it along on our vacation. I'll read it aloud in the car.

Once, after a bitter fight, Mike asked me if I was capable
of loving someone with more conservative views than I held.
(While Mike will not say he is conservative, he will admit to
being more conservative than I am.) Could I still like him? I
did not answer.

I thought about it awhile and later in bed I said what I'd
heard people say. "I think the most important thing is that
we both have the same values," I ventured, testing it out on
myself as well as him.

An older female friend of mine had told me that people
don't separate over politics. Her husband, for example, thinks
abortion is murder. (I know I couldn't take that.) She said
couples split over the "important things": disagreements about
child-raising, money, where they want to live. Mike and I are
childless, don't have enough money to argue over, and can't
move until he gets out of school. More importantly, we are
not married and have not decided we want to be. That subject
is one we do not address, during an argument or at any other
time. Perhaps my mother was right. Not that I consider our
political disagreements irrelevant, but what we do *not* debate
may be as revealing as what we do. Mike and I argue about
everything except whether we are fit for each other. That
discussion could topple the structure we have so carefully con-
structed: Laurie and Mike, the free-standing couple. Together,

they explore faraway places, they work hard, they scorn pretension in the way that all born-and-bred Midwesterners do.

We are both getting older, each privately considering the prospect of settling down with the other, and in so many ways we seem an ideal match. We like the idea of Laurie and Mike. For now, we want it, we want us, to work. And so we don't dare discuss the big question and the differences rumbling beneath the surface that may make it impossible to commit to a future together. Since we are not ready to consider razing what we've built, well, we're still going at it.

"Laurie," Mike groans, "I'm only saying that in the end antidiscrimination laws may do more harm than good."

"That's fine for you," I shoot back, "but you've obviously never been black or a woman."

Dancing

MAGDA KRANCE

Before lust knows what it is, it finds its first awkward expression in dancing. It's almost innocent then (though it urgently doesn't want to be), as it blindly gropes toward—what it isn't yet sure.

Junior-high dances were like that, all tingly with presexual longing and sweet anxiety. Is anyone going to ask me to dance? Will it be one of the guys I *like*? Will he put *both* arms around me during a slow song? Does that mean he *likes* me? And what does *that* mean? This was in mid-sixties middle

America, a proverbial Time of Innocence, before preteens got pregnant on an alarmingly regular basis. My girlfriends and I longed to become the images we pored over in *Seventeen*— cool teenage sophisticates at coed parties with clever themes, daughters of mothers who served delicious-sounding snacks and then disappeared. Instead, we were gangly, clumsy, stumbling, shuffling tomboys in sheepish clothing, gathered in corners and giggling nervously in our school gym with its homely, earnest decorations. We were nothing like the snappy, sexy types that filled the dance floor on *American Bandstand*.

But even tomboys can have moments of raw sexiness. I was thirteen, and had ridden my bike to a summer girlfriend's place a mile away. We were listening to a song by the Association that was uncharacteristically sexy, and we were prancing about like mad in our little-girl bikinis—shimmying as erotically as we knew how, which wasn't very, yet. Still, when Sue's father walked in on us, all three of us became a little flustered and embarrassed. A stunned look washed over his face—he seemed genuinely startled at the inevitable metamorphosis of two budding nymphettes and, perhaps, at his own arousal, though none of this occurred to me until years later.

By sixteen, my dance-floor technique had blossomed, along with my sexuality. I could gyrate and hip-thrust provocatively, and I enjoyed the attention I knew my dancing could generate. That year, I spent a heady summer vacation in France, traveling all by myself from one set of family friends to another. At one point I was in a resort disco with a French girlfriend; each of us was being hit on by some sleazy local. As mine held me too close, he whispered, "Zee slow dahnceeng ees a verticahl pozeetion fohr a hohreezontahl deesire." I was somewhat grossed out as I tried to squirm out of his tightening grasp, but the truism never left me. With the right partner on the right dance floor, it's a wonderful turn-on of a line.

At its best, dancing is the consummate expression of word-less desire, unrequited love, unbridled horniness, longed-for consummation, and love achieved. It is terrifically revealing of who we are, who we want to be, and how we want to be seen. It is flirtation made physical, the foreplay to foreplay. It can be simultaneously innocent and sordid, safe and smol-dering, public and very private. It can be a simple celebration of individual physicality, a joyous, exuberant romp that has nothing to do with sex.

For all those reasons, it can also be terribly misunderstood. Dancing can be downright dangerous. It can lead to devasta-ting misunderstandings, date rape, and worse.

When I was nineteen, I lived in Greece on a semester-abroad program. My folk-dance class took a field trip to a tiny northern village unknown to tourists, where each year's pre-Lent carnival is marked by wild street dancing. Troupes of villagers clad in shaggy goatskin costumes banged drums, brandished wooden swords, swilled tiny bottles of banana-flavored rotgut, and danced all day in a primal, centuries-old ritual. We watched, enchanted and fascinated. That night, I joined a group of my teachers in a taverna, where they were sitting with a group of local shepherds. Together they formed a *pareia*, a clique, and by joining them I became part of it, although I didn't realize it.

When a man from another table, another *pareia*, asked me to join a circle dance, I eagerly accepted, not because I found him attractive (I didn't), but because I figured this was a great way to practice what I'd learned in the classroom, and show off for my teachers. Unknown to me, this offended my *pareia*, but they let it pass because I was an ignorant young American, after all.

Then the band began to play a *tsifteteli*, a very suggestive one-on-one belly dance. Again, eager to show off my dancing prowess, I began shimmying with abandon. Suddenly one of my teachers grabbed me and slammed me into a chair. "Don't

move!" she ordered. "Our" shepherds rushed out on the street
with the *pareia* of the man who had asked me to dance, angrily
talking guns and knives, threatening each other. His wife had
happened to show up while we were dancing, got upset, and
was fully ready to kill me herself. The shepherds were poised
to do battle to defend me. Somehow, the situation was de-
fused, and we left unscathed. Later, one of the teachers told
me she'd never seen sociosexual ethics laid out so clearly.
Indeed.

Back in America, I had a better grasp of the ground rules.
The summer I was twenty, I started dating a guy I'd known
casually in high school. Back then, I had made fun of the way
he played jazz saxophone; with all that soulful pelvis thrusting,
why didn't he just turn his horn around, hmmmm? Now,
I had a new appreciation for what had seemed silly before.
His hips and limbs churned and pushed like muscular pis-
tons, somehow both precise and spontaneous. He danced
with a ripened but playful erotic intensity, enhanced by his
musician's sense of rhythm and improvisation. Wonderfully,
in short.

One night that summer, we went to a tacky bar in our
hometown, a place I'd never been to before and have never
been to since. We were deliciously carnal in our dancing. Our
hips would graze, then grind. A breathless bimbette simpered
away from her partner and sidled up to me. "Is that your
boyfriend? Jeez, he dances good!" "Yesss," I hissed smugly,
thinking to myself, "And he's mine, all mine!" A few weeks
later, I accompanied him back to his university, which resumed classes a few weeks before mine did. My last night in
town we went dancing. We jumped and bumped and rubbed
in a sweaty, beery, horny, end-of-summer, classes-are-about-
to-start frenzy along with what felt like thousands of other
students packed into a cavernous college bar, all of us verti-
cally driving at horizontality. A few hours later, pedal to the
metal, we arrived.

Everything changed just one year later, when I went to a close friend's wedding in northern Minnesota. That night, at the wedding dance at the township meeting hall, I remet my future husband, with whom the bride and I had gone to college. (She'd lived with him romantically in a communal house; when things fell apart, she moved in with me.) Steve wasn't exactly dazzling on the dance floor; in fact, his moves were a bit peculiar. There was something about him, though, that transcended that point. In time, we got around to dating, courting, and marrying. Once, out dancing with a bunch of others, I commented on Steve's odd dance style to another guy. "And you know what's beautiful about him? He doesn't care!" our friend said with genuine admiration and appreciation.

For me, dancing is so closely tied to lust and flirtation that there's no real place for it in my life anymore. At the occasional wedding we still dance, of course. We do it well, in our own way, and we still enjoy it, but it no longer has the burning, defining urgency for me that it once did. The need to act on that horizontal desire is no longer driven by its being illicit. With our desires sanctioned by marriage, there are other ways and places beyond the exhibitionism of the dance floor.

LOVESTRUCK

Fidelity

JANICE ROSENBERG

At a party on a ski trip, a man in my ski class, a man whom I'd been flirting with all week, asked me to dance. Or maybe I asked him. My husband had gone off to dance with one of the single women in our class (so that she wouldn't feel left out, he told me later), leaving me at the table with this man I'd wanted to be alone with for days.

Whose ever idea it was, we ended up dancing. The band played a ballad. I stopped short of telling him that what I really wanted was to sleep with him, and that I considered dancing the next best thing. Instead I told him that we were dancing just the way I'd always wanted to dance. He looked at me as if he thought I was deranged, which at the time I was. What I meant had nothing to do with the ordinary way our feet were moving and everything to do with our proximity.

My husband and I had met this man the first afternoon of our vacation. After spending a morning trying to ski on our own—befuddled by the German signs in the Swiss ski resort and discouraged by the steep mountaintop ski runs—we noticed a class on a miniature hill behind a hotel in town. We asked the teacher to let us join. We were beginners with just enough experience to match his morning's lesson, so we fit right in.

The man I later danced with quickly made friends with us. I assumed that he viewed friendship with a couple the easiest way to protect himself from predatory single women in the class. He was a New Yorker, the kind you associated with the Upper West Side or Brooklyn Heights, civilized. He knew the score. Over the course of a sunny afternoon sidestepping up the incline and waiting for our turns at skiing down, we three determined how nearly our opinions meshed on half a dozen subjects.

In no time, I developed a terrific crush on the man. It's not bad to have a crush on someone if you know that's what it is and can laugh at yourself. But if you think it means that you have to sleep with him, or that you'll never get over him, and you're also married, a crush can create problems. That week in Switzerland I not only had those notions, I reveled in them.

I've thought a lot about why I needed those particular sensations at that point in my life. I now know my infatuation was no accident. I cultivated my feelings, minimal at first, into the storm that followed and somehow saw the entire episode as something I deserved. Why did I do this?

I'd rarely had the opportunity to test my sex appeal as an adult woman with an adult man. This man was older, worldly. He found my obvious interest flattering, knew the game, and played it just well enough to keep me going. For an entire week I operated on two levels. I was misbehaving and knew it. I did nothing to stop myself. I was miserable; I really did care for this man, wanted to run off with him. At the same time, I saw the whole event as a melodrama. A skier on a too-hard run, I had declared myself out of control: everyone else had better watch out. At the same time, I was manipulative, egging my husband on to new heights of jealousy that culminated in his saying back home that if I ever acted that way again, he'd kill me.

Eventually I unknotted this tangled mess. I admitted to

myself that my fascination with the New York skier had little to do with *his* attributes and everything to do with my self-esteem or lack thereof. I was twenty-five, had just had a baby, wanted someone—a man—to convince me that I was still attractive, that I was smart and clever and looked good on skis. Near the end of the week, the man remarked to my husband that I was a "live wire." I took it as a compliment, thinking he meant that I was scintillating. More likely he meant that I was sparking near combustible material, dangerous and in need of expert handling.

That was twenty years ago. Since then I've learned that crushes don't have to be painful. For a couple of months now I've had what I think of as a sensible crush on an aerobics instructor named David. If he's as old as thirty, I'll eat my spandex pedal-pushers. If he's even twenty-five. He's handsome, muscular, with a big smile full of white teeth. With his baseball cap on backwards, he's adorable. My husband and I joke about my Sunday-morning meetings with David. I look forward to seeing him at a distance for an hour once a week. He's literally on a stage. I don't talk to him. I sometimes imagine what it would be like to share an afternoon in bed with him. All things being equal, why not check it out? My body's okay, and I know what I'm doing in bed. With David I could probably handle my emotions, keep the encounter strictly at the level of amusement.

All this came to mind as I listened to a married friend describe the crush she had on a man she'd met in a neighborhood volunteer group. Her definition of a crush fell somewhere between the two styles I've described. She insisted that she loved her husband and that kissing and necking with this man was just for fun. She wasn't in love with the guy, didn't plan to be. She simply had a crush on him and saw nothing wrong with acting on it. How far that "acting" would go she couldn't say. Circumstances and available time would govern that. I pictured her checking her watch over his shoulder as they kissed.

I listened to her with mixed emotions. Mostly I was amazed that she could be involved with another man, and reveal nothing about that involvement at home either accidentally or accidentally-on-purpose. She seemed able to compartmentalize her life, to keep one section from bleeding into the other. She loved her husband. She was only fooling around with this guy. I admired her self-control and at the same time shivered at her coolness.

Her stories, I admit, gave me a bit of a vicarious thrill. As she spoke, I imagined myself necking in a cloakroom with a handsome stranger. I imagined just as easily the panic I'd feel facing my husband if he ever found out and the chagrin I'd feel living with myself even if he didn't. My friend stated absolutely that her husband would not find out, and that if he did, she didn't think it would be so bad. After all, hadn't she told him when he went on a recent business trip to a city where an old girlfriend lived that he should enjoy himself, but practice safe sex? Didn't that establish *their* intention to have what was called—in that misguided 1970s fad—an "open marriage"?

Did her husband get the hint? I wondered. Listening to her tale, I couldn't help thinking about him. Did he assume that she was perfectly faithful? Would he consider her kissing another man okay within the framework of their marriage? I suppose some couples have worked that out, but I can't help thinking that no matter how suave they try to be, one or the other always ends up hurt.

My friend's story unfolded over a number of weeks. Never once did she mention feeling guilty. Nor did she admit being frightened of discovery or of what that discovery might do to her marriage. I listened without comment because I didn't want to sound judgmental, prissy, self-righteous, or envious.

I felt uncomfortable, like a parent who hears that someone else's kid is taking drugs and doesn't try to stop him.

Finally, I told her that I didn't approve. I was careful not to soften or qualify my statement with phrases like "I know this is going to sound old-fashioned, but . . ." or "I know I'm just a little bit envious, but . . ." or "I hope you don't mind my saying so, but . . ." I wanted my comment to have its full effect so I just said it straight out: "I disapprove."

She said she knew and understood. What she was doing wasn't for everyone, she said, the implication being that I was meek and cowed, domesticated, bourgeois, maybe just a little bit undersexed, while she was bold and brave, a risk-taker formed in a different mold. She said she needed more excitement in her life than one steady man provided. Her logic followed the cheater's age-old pattern: "I need this. I can handle this. Therefore, I'll have this."

It's impossible to talk about adultery—let's go ahead and say the ugly word—without getting on a soapbox, so here I go. Lying and secrets don't fit with marriage. Honesty and openness do. Marriage is a social contract, which means that you give up certain things to get certain others. You give up sexual variety for the satisfaction of knowing someone inside out. You give up discovering new partners for the surprise of discovering new depths in the person whom you know best. You give up flaunting your outward allure for the pleasure of knowing that there is much more of value to you than what meets the eye.

So much for lectures. Now I'll speak about myself. The world's a complex, confusing place. I need something steady in the center, and for me that steady center is my marriage. Living fully in it, I share companionship, comfort, sex, love, hugs, acceptance, friendship, sympathy, support, thoughtful criticism, honest compliments, children, common history, and laughter. I can depend on having all that and more. Things that are dependable need not be boring. My life still has its highs and lows and complications.

The complications caused by sex with another man, even if that "sex" is limited to a kiss or two, are not the complications that I want. If I had the circumstances of the Swiss trip to replay (which, in a grander sense, it occurs to me, I *do* have all the time), if everything were the same except that I was the me that I am now, my husband and I, as a pair, would offer that man our friendship and company. That man (I hope) would find me charming, funny, at ease with myself and with my decision to remain faithfully married to my husband.

I would certainly consider him attractive, sophisticated, and urbane. I would no doubt feel a measure of wistfulness knowing that I would never have him for a lover. As compensation for this loss, I would be able to enjoy him as a person and be satisfied to know the feeling was returned—something I couldn't do when he was the object of that perilous crush.

I've made an active choice to be faithful, not just in spirit like my friend, but to the letter. I think that at some point, every woman who remains faithful to her husband has to make that choice and has to continue making it on a regular basis.

Younger Men

LAURIE ABRAHAM

Feeling the need to converse with some like-minded souls and perhaps to flirt with some like-minded men, I decided to attend a discussion on the media coverage of the Persian Gulf War. It was a sure bet, I thought. Packed with liberal magazine editors, the panel promised a cozy refuge from the cold, cruel conservative world. It was sure to be a case of the panel preaching to the converted, but that was fine by me. I wanted to be among the converted. So off I went to the café—appropriately named the "Hot House"—wearing a short, rather clingy cinnamon-colored dress, black tights, and black cowboy boots. Come hither, liberals, my outfit beckoned.

The talk was already under way when I arrived, so I stood in the door and surveyed the scene. Gathered around small tables, the audience was listening attentively: one gray head, a white one, a black tam, a salt-and-pepper beard. Not an under-forty face in the lot, it seemed. Sadly for the future of progressive politics, as well as for my own social future, a conservative subject like "How the Media Helped Saddam Hussein Almost Win the War" probably would have drawn a younger crowd. Whereas the people assembled here were still fighting for social change, their care-worn faces showed defeat, or more likely just the effects of families and nine-to-five jobs. Whatever the cause, they were hardly flirting material.

It turned out that the talk had attracted a few Communists, who railed on and on in dated clichés, refusing to give up the floor to other speakers. But one participant stood out: One of the few men in the room under fifty, he had a backpack slung over his shoulder, and his question was the first of the question-and-answer period. And it was thoughtful. The panelists responded in kind, but the respite was short-lived. As yet another harangue began, I got up to leave. Striding out of the room in my new cowboy boots—I might as well have worn penny loafers—I stopped at the bar for a beer.

The talk broke up, and the questioner came and stood near me. He ordered a coffee. I felt his presence. It was jittery, coltish. I kept my back to him out of nervousness, which too often overcomes me when I can tell a man wants to introduce himself to me. He took the plunge anyway. "How did you like the talk?" he asked.

Well, that was all I needed. I launched into my own harangue about the Communists' harangues, and he nodded in agreement. Then we asked about each other. The backpack was for real; he was a senior at the journalism school that I had graduated from five years before. That made him about twenty-two. I told him my name and he recognized it. He actually read the race and poverty publication for which I was a reporter. I could see that he was impressed. He wanted to work at an "alternative" paper, too. "Like yours," he said. He managed to slip into the conversation the fact that he was one of the founders of a new campus magazine that had won a national award, beating out entries from Harvard and the like. He also had interned at *The New Republic*, so I was impressed. But what was so remarkable was that he was more impressed by my story than I was by his. I was the working journalist; I had something he wanted—connections and some power in the "alternative" publications world. He was still a student.

Scenes from the movie *White Palace*, about a fortyish

woman and a man my age who fall in love, rolled through
my mind. The movie was as much about class differences as
about May-September romances, but it had charmed me and
piqued my curiosity about dating younger men. The reasons
women usually give for dating younger men are that they are
less sexist and more energetic. Qualities like these are only
revealed over the course of a relationship, so they did not have
much to do with my attraction to the journalism student, Ned.
What seduced me was the potential for power: my power over
him.

He was witty and smart but just beginning to search for
his place in the writing world. I imagined him wanting me
not for my femininity (though I certainly had not kept it under
wraps that night) but for my clout. He might want to use me
to get to the top, I thought. What a rush! It was intoxicating
to have something a man wanted from me more than he
wanted sex. For a few delectable moments, the relationship
between the sexes was turned upside down.

Of course, I hope and trust that my male friends are interested in my knowledge and companionship more than my sex,
but that is irrelevant. I am not talking about friendships; I am
discussing first-time encounters between women and men,
what attracts men and women to each other. Sure, men today
increasingly choose women for what they do, but how they
look still takes precedence, and the reverse is true for women.
This is nothing shocking or new, and not precisely what I am
talking about, either. Ned did not tantalize me simply because
he was a reporter. The point is that I could make something
happen for him, which is a power I have thus far not had
much chance to wield.

Ned's youthfulness gave this meeting its special charm, as
I'm typically not drawn to men less successful than I. Perhaps
that makes me sound like what one friend would call a "power
fucker," but I do not think that label fits me (perhaps it doesn't
fit many women; perhaps it's a tag stuck on women by inse-

cure men). My respect for men and women alike is in large measure based on what they do and how well they do it. That was what was so ideal about Ned; he obviously had a great future in front of him, he had potential, but he was not there yet. I could help him get there. (Maybe, after all, I just wanted to mother him. . . . No!)

I suppose that some people, especially men, will be offended by such a bald discussion of power in love relationships between women and men. "These are the nineties—doesn't she believe in equality?" some men will no doubt complain. That reaction reminds me of an encounter I witnessed at a workshop on race relations.

"I am color-blind," a white minister told a black man. There was a long pause.

"Maybe you have the luxury to be color-blind, but I don't," the black man retorted. "I'm forced to think about what color I am every time I walk out the door." And, the man continued, someone who's color-blind denies a central part of his existence, being black. In other words, it's easy to be color-blind when you're the right color. I say something similar to men who scoff at my unseemly talk of power: It's easy to be power-blind when you've got it.

But let me get on with my fantasy. For days, I thought about this Ned, imagined taking him around to meet my reporter friends, sharing beers with him, visiting his collegiate apartment. For the record, I didn't imagine sleeping with him; for some reason, I have difficulty fantasizing about having sex with someone I've never had sex with. Then one morning, I flipped on the radio. And there was Ned. He was being interviewed on National Public Radio about an article he had written that past summer for a national magazine. I had been interviewed on local public radio, but never national. I couldn't believe it was him.

The magic was gone.

Fear of Romance

LAURA GREEN

I want to win a million dollars. I would like to be twenty knowing what I know now. I am dying to go to Kenya and see a rhino on the slopes of Mount Meru or Kilimanjaro. I wish I were romantic.

I used to believe I hated romance because it was phony. Romance held up relationships that should collapse. It was a potion people swallowed to fall in love. Romance, I argued, is what they used in ads to sell you cigarettes and weekend hotel packages. But the truth is that I hated romance the way some girls hate prom queens—out of simple, frustrated envy. I am jealous of romantics. They know how to lose themselves in the moment and have fun. They make people feel good. They can enjoy their money, and they love to dance. I want to be like that. I want my husband to be that way, too, even though I tell myself that two romantics under one roof would go bankrupt.

It isn't as if I have never done romantic things. I once stood in the most beautiful place I ever saw, a field in northern California. It was filled with flowering lupines and at its center was a spreading live oak. So many bumblebees buzzed around the lupines that the air was filled with their humming. Though I had never seen that field before and will probably never find it again, I recognized it. When I was a little girl, it was the field I imagined when I read about meadows in storybooks.

I once went swimming in a pool in the mountains of West Africa at dusk, with a crescent moon rising. I have walked through Venice in the rain. But I did these things alone, or with friends, so their romance is the romance of travel, not of love.

It is easy to confuse travel, romance, and love. For someone like me, who yearns to be romantic and doesn't know how, the results can be disastrous.

One winter, shortly after my first marriage ended, a man I was dating asked me to go to Mexico with him. If I would pick up the cost of my flight, he said, he would do the rest. He had recently separated from his wife and I think he needed moral support. I admired him tremendously. Talented, hip, witty, respected, and on top of things, he was everything I wanted to be (except that I didn't want to be male, of course).

Vulnerable, hurt, unaware that we were entering an all-or-nothing situation, we plunged into the most romantic setting I ever saw. It was perfect for a honeymoon—if you didn't mind the caretaker wandering over for a joint late in the afternoon. The vacation house, a white, flower-covered cottage with a long veranda that overlooked the Pacific, was on a very private bay near Acapulco, part of a compound of five or six houses that spilled down a steep hill in a shower of bougainvillea, iguanas, stucco, red brick ledges, and blue, blue swimming pools. At one end of our villa's pool grew a mango tree whose leaves hung so low they nearly brushed the water. I loved to dive in, swim underwater through blazing blue so bright I could almost see through my shut eyelids, then shoot up into the dark green leaves. Bursting from the water, naked and clean, rising from the light into the blackness of the leaves, grabbing a mango, was the most exhilarating thing I ever did. If only I could have translated that into romance.

The memory of it still thrills me but it is the thrill of the cold water, the blinding sun, and the intense color. It had everything to do with the setting and very little to do with the man I had come with. We were not in love and the romantic setting was a rebuke. It didn't have to be that way, but I wanted to be head over heels and nothing else. If only I had just let myself be seduced! If only he had had the energy to do it.

On paper, the match should have worked. We were in the same business. We had similar tastes, or rather, his taste was exquisite and I was trying hard to catch up. We were into a talky, finger-popping urbanity. But there was little chemistry between us and no romance for a catalyst.

I tried hard. So did he. During the day, we swam in the clear cove and watched tropical fish browse around the underwater boulders and sprawled together under palm-frond shelters at the beach. We wandered through the open-air market and bought trinkets. In the evening, we sat in butterfly chairs on the terrace watching the sun light every pink, Rubenesque curve of the clouds that rolled above our heads, opening, closing, and merging like the most sensuous bodies. But once the sun had set in a last brassy flare along the Pacific and it was too cold to swim, and too late to go into town for the movie, I lost my nerve. Night brought awkward silences over drinks that got warm. We fumbled about in bed and apologized to each other afterwards.

If only he had asked me to dance on the terrace. If only I could have taken his hand and led him there. We didn't need to fall in love; we just needed to have fun. If only we had been flexible enough to give in to a setting where every tree, every terrace, every flower said, "This is made for romance."

When the week was up, we both were glad to go home. The tension of wondering why we weren't swept away by Mexico had been exhausting. I think I talked to him once or twice after that. Looking for love and unwilling to find romance, I ruined a perfectly fine friendship.

A year after my Acapulco fiasco, the spring before we got married, my husband and I decided to drive through northern Ontario, the kind of decision made by fools in love. It is freezing there in June, and the black flies swarm by the millions, stinging everything warm-blooded and driving the moose so crazy they run out onto the highways and into the paths of the few cars on the road. Floating along on a pheromone tide, or whatever it is that arouses us sexually, I would have followed my love into a burning building.

We drove through a desolate, intimidating, beautiful region of abandoned farmsteads, old beaver meadows covered with blue iris, and endless cedar swamps. It was like a honeymoon in the Yukon, so cold we were barely able to get near one another's skin. The itchy layers of the wool we wore most of the time were bad enough, but we also had to rub a greasy citronella compound into our faces, hair, and hands to keep the black flies away. We lived out of a musty little tent and my ancient Chevy, which had 120,000 miles on it, cooked outdoors, and stank of smoke and insect repellent. The dark and dreary evenings in our smelly tent were the antithesis of Acapulco sunsets. The only people we saw were hippies from Glasgow and Cree Indians from Hudson Bay. Both the Indians and the Scots spoke an English so different from ours as to make conversation almost impossible. We were thrown into each other's arms by the cold, and into each other's thoughts by the utter lack of diversion. By the time we headed home, we both knew, without discussing it, that we would get married.

No one would have called it romantic, but I was in love and that compensated. Still, given my choice, I would rather have gone to Acapulco with my husband and been miserable in Ontario with someone else. I want to hold my husband's hand while watching the sunset over the Pacific. He is the one who should go swimming with me in Africa. Cut adrift from the telephone and deadlines, I would like to believe, we will dance on a hundred terraces. Slow music will play and we will feel it rather than hear it.

I am dreaming. We don't dance much and when we do, we are awkward. He snaps his fingers and waves his hands; I shuffle and bite my lip. I know that if only we could waltz, it would be the key that unlocks us. Dancing and romance are linked. If you can let go for one, you will not turn your back on the other. Romantics don't worry what other people think. They are not inhibited. They would never say, "It's too expensive," or "I feel silly," the things I have said hoping that my husband would talk me out of them.

I have been lucky. I have love. But, given the choice between love's permanence and romance's evanescence, I would choose both. I would like to walk down the narrow streets of Venice with my husband, my arm around his waist and his around mine, aware of every step, of each stony archway, of the smells, the sea beyond, ready to float into a dream of romance.

Reflections on Romance

I've got a love-hate, approach-avoidance relationship with the whole notion of romance and its many trappings. I scorn it and shun it, but also yearn for it, at least a little. I can be unabashedly sexual and sexy, but the whole idea of romance makes me squeamish.

Romance eludes clear definition. To me, the words "romance" and "romantic" conjure up a collage of glossy images, predominantly from television, magazines, and movies: slender, elegantly dressed lovers with perfect teeth whirling across a dance floor, or laughing into the wind at the rail of a luxury liner, or gazing deeply into each other's sparkling eyes over a sumptuous dinner, or sipping champagne while lounging in a Jacuzzi. They do not have bad breath. They do not burp or fart or sweat. They do not have bits of food caught between their perfect teeth. They do not have stretch marks or unsightly hair. They do not interrupt each other. They do not yawn. They are, in short, not human.

This is not my life, or, presumably, anyone else's, but these are the hackneyed images that swim into mind at the mention of things romantic. I can't help it. My own possibly romantic visions are eclipsed by that commercialized clutter. I can't seem to elbow my way into those mass-media images of romantic perfection.

Take, for instance, the night my husband and I spent at a bed-and-breakfast in Minnesota. The place had a double Jacuzzi tub and fireplace in every room—the interior-design iconography of romance. We used the sunken bath self-consciously, mainly out of a sense of obligation for having paid for it. It felt more silly than romantic, because it just wasn't the kind of thing we *do*. What does stand out in my memory, though, is the guestbook in the room, in which previous occupants had recorded their romantic impressions of that particular room ("The night was cold! The tub and sex were hot!" and many far worse). I'm no prude, but I was grossed out. I was having a hard enough time feeling romantic on my own, and I didn't want the ghosts of other people's intimacy staining the sheets and muddying the waters, as they were in my imagination. I know; I could have put the book down, but I was morbidly fascinated by the awful inscriptions.

Romance is a minefield of implications and expectations. For it to be too important would be both dangerous and disappointing. For it to be entirely absent would make life mighty dull. Romance is like perfume—an enhancer, an attention-getter, an intoxicant for the emotions, a catalyst for things to come. Or is that lust I'm describing? It's not always easy to tell them apart. Love, sex, lust, and romance tend to get inextricably intertwined, like colors in a painter's palette or ingredients in a complex sauce. Definitions are elusive. Whatever it is, one whiff can stop me in my tracks, nostrils flared, ears perked, skin tingling, muscles tensed, eyes scanning alertly for the source.

Not that that has happened lately. In my current life, I'm contentedly married and maternal, both for the long haul. I now work full-time—the possibility of a midday quickie no longer exists in the way it did when we both worked at home. In our time together we take care of our son, run errands, bike, windsurf, cook, watch the news, read the papers, and fall asleep. Our lives are pretty well saturated. There isn't much time or appetite for major romantic activity right now. To extend a simile from a few lines back, I don't use perfume much anymore, either—most days and nights, it just doesn't occur to me. It's the stuff of special dress-up occasions now. The tiny half-full bottles that still crowd my dresser are souvenirs of an earlier life that needed that sensory accessory more often. These days, I'm grateful to get into the shower every few days.

Having said that, however, we have recently rediscovered the pleasure of going on a regular date with each other—dinner, movie, holding hands, exchanging warm glances, talking at length without the usual interruptions (not during the movie, of course). Seduction isn't the point of these occasional evenings, though—just enjoying each other's company is, outside of the context of the usual responsibilities.

Earlier in my married life, I flirted promiscuously. I seemed to need more approval and appraisal then, more romance or possibility of romance, perhaps, and I found it in lingering glances and flashy conversations with other men. It was fun; it was risky, off-limits behavior (a bit of danger is a terrific romance enhancer), and it made me feel good. I always came home invigorated, and Steve was the beneficiary. I would feel a different kind of energy and excitement, as if my return to him were a first encounter.

What is romantic? For me, it's a gesture or an evanescent moment born of surprise and imagination, something that leaves me breathless and giddy and flushed with love or lust, or both. Breaking the barrier between interest and passion—the hand tentatively touching the knee, the first quivering kiss, and all that follows—is the essence of romance. But so is impulsively wedging into the same compartment of a revolving door at a bank, stopping halfway through, laughing and making out for a few minutes in full view of amused passersby, something that happened a long, long time ago. And so is an unexpected kiss on the back of the neck, a spontaneous shared laugh that lights our eyes, a slightly salacious grazing of our bodies as we pass in our daily chores—those are the proverbial embers of our romance in our day-to-day lives, and they still warm.

Certainly I've been in love (and in lust), and certainly I've reveled in romantic moments and gestures. I've pined and moped over an unrequited love in the manner of a true romantic. On the other hand, I came of age at a time when women weren't supposed to need romance. By the time I got to college in the early 1970s, my peers and I were budding feminists. We proclaimed ourselves liberated. If we wanted to make love or have sex, we did it without needing to be buttered up with dopey romantic gestures. Accordingly, the guys we saw (not "dated") were wary of making those gestures, afraid of being called sexist pigs or worse.

When Steve and I were courting, just out of college, we were both rather hippieish and practical, more inclined to industrial-strength cotton briefs and undershirts than to sexy lingerie, which, after all, was regarded at the time as a blatant symbol of oppression. It was not politically correct for it to play a part in relationships. In any case, our ardor never seemed to need the props. On the rare occasion, though, when I would put up with the discomfort of some teasing little undergarment, he always discovered it with surprised pleasure.

It might be different now, if I were dating, as far as lingerie is concerned. I might want to be a package waiting to be unwrapped, bursting with frilly and enticing surprises, something different each time. But probably not. I don't think it's in my nature. Once in a very rare while, I dig through my dresser drawers to find something more suggestive and seductive, to conform as best as I can to the Victoria's Secret mail-order image of romance, but I usually feel a little self-conscious and contrived doing so and tend to change back into something more comfortable and utilitarian as soon as it's tactful.

Were we ever romantic in those standardized, conventional ways? Not really, though there have been some sweet and glorious moments. When we were in our early twenties, Steve asked me to live with him by shyly giving me a set of towels for our new apartment and a homely bouquet of limp spring wildflowers he'd picked in a forest preserve—hardly a conventionally lavish romantic overture, but it was straight from his heart, and true to his north-woods practical nature. (We still have the towels, which by this time are fairly tattered, but sentimentality keeps me from using them as rags.) When we were nearly ten years married he surprised me with a gorgeous band of gold and diamonds for my birthday—yep, just like in the "diamonds are forever" ads.

I did have major romantic expectations for a wedding proposal. I was sure he would pop the question on a mountaintop in the Adirondacks. Oblivious to my certainty, he didn't. Or when we canoed in northern Minnesota—surely the rustic setting was a perfect counterpoint for the engagement ring I imagined he would fetch from some inner jacket pocket. My vividly choreographed romantic fantasy remained just that.

When the right time came, the decision to marry occurred spontaneously to both of us in the afterglow of afternoon lovemaking on the floor-bound mattress that nearly filled our tiny post-collegiate bedroom. It was, in retrospect, a wonderfully romantic moment, and distinctively, quirkily ours. After we proposed to each other, we rolled out of bed, set up a camera on a tripod, sat on our dumpy sofa looking dreamily at each other, and recorded the moment for posterity—and our unconventional wedding announcement. Many of our peers were shocked—shocked!—at my unbuttoned shirt, Steve's bare chest, and our telltale sex flush, obvious even in the black-and-white photograph. Most of my mother's friends, ironi-

cally, were delighted and amused, finding in the image, perhaps, an echo of my parents' younger years.

I grew up in a home filled with the romantic piano music
of Chopin and Brahms, played by my father, who loved life
deeply and who died at the age of sixty-one, when I was
eighteen. He was a wonderfully European gentleman (although not stuffy or snobby) whose every gesture seemed utterly exotic and romantic to his American acquaintances. The
fact that he could just sit down and play these heartbreakingly
beautiful nocturnes and ballades made him an inspiring and
romantic figure in the eyes of all who knew him. He and my
mother absolutely adored each other, a wonderful and rare
thing that I took for granted as a child. They kissed and embraced and laughed and frequently shared looks of deep love.
In old photographs and in my memory, they seemed the em-
bodiment of both romantic and settled love, always beaming
and bright-eyed and mischievous, as if they shared a wonderful secret—which of course they did. Yet my father was also
a consummate flirt, kissing the hands of his friends' wives and
making them feel wonderfully wanted without making the
men feel threatened or my mother feel the least bit jealous or
unappreciated.

My parents' torch was passed, at least aspects of it. I like
to believe our marriage is a reasonable parallel to theirs, replete
with love and fun and contentment, secure enough to allow a
bit of recreational flirtation. Maybe it's even romantic occasionally—in its own way.

Romance I

LAURIE ABRAHAM

Many of my women friends suspect romance, scorn it as a contrivance, or wrinkle their noses and say flowers, candy, and golden sunsets turn their stomachs. This happened again a few nights ago when one of my closest friends came to dinner. Before Lana arrived, it occurred to me that I'd created a rather romantic setting for our meal. The table glittered; I'd draped a runner over it, a luxuriant length of fabric shot with silver and gold. On top of that I'd placed a small candle in a crystal holder. I kept the lights low and switched on a Lava lamp my boyfriend had given me. Corny and dated, maybe, but Lava lamps give a dimly lit room a mysterious, dreamy quality; the scarlet liquid hovers in the gold like bunchy red storm clouds. The point is I like to create moods, build sets for the small dramas of my life. And with Lana's lover out of town for the weekend, I'd planned—without really thinking about it—an evening of intimacy, of sharing confidences with a friend.

Midway through dinner, I told Lana what I thought was a delectable story about another friend whose boyfriend fed her strawberries in the bathtub to celebrate her return home from a business trip. Lana laughed and the topic changed, but a few minutes later, she told me that though berries in the bath sounded sweet in one way, in another, the whole thing sounded "*disgusting*." It seemed so artificial, she went on. If any man pulled a stunt like that with her, she would think he'd lost his mind. She shifted uncomfortably in her chair, imagining the scene. Lana is warm, laughs easily, and gets a bit raucous every once in a while; all by way of saying, she's not a bore. And as I've mentioned, I've heard other friends express sentiments similar to hers. I'm the one who's out of sync here: As soon as I heard the strawberry story, I planned to repeat it to my lover, hoping that he might feed me someday.

That suggests perhaps the fundamental difference between my attitude toward romance and my friends'. It doesn't matter to me whether the champagne's been poured before, whether other couples have embraced on the ship's deck gazing at an orange sunset, or fallen together into a four-poster bed at a country inn. I don't care if men through the ages (through the advertising ages, even) have given women jewels in tiny blue velvet boxes in front of crackling fires. The standard romantic repertoire has been played thousands of times before, and I love it all the same.

I appreciate equally the unexpected gesture, the quirky romantic moment. I remember Mike pulling off to the side of the freeway, grabbing my hand, and pulling me over a grassy embankment. We made love there, barely concealed, with the semis roaring by. This past summer, when I was having a particularly bad day, he went to the Art Institute during his lunch hour and bought me a Gauguin poster to brighten my home office. I picked up the phone recently and heard "our song" playing. We live a thousand miles apart now, and he did not say one word until the song was over. By that time, I was crying. Each of these experiences sparkled with romance, of an original, impromptu variety.

But I am not about to leave romance to chance, or completely in his hands. Part of the thrill comes from the expectation. When I was a child, I tried to wait until the last possible

moment to open my Christmas presents. I exclaimed enthusi-
astically over my sister's gifts, my mother's, hoping that if
they were occupied admiring their own loot, they would forget about handing wrapped boxes to me. When I finally had
to give in, I pulled off the foil paper ever so slowly, one bit
of tape, then another and another. The high of anticipation is
one of the parts of a long-distance relationship that I appreciate
and sometimes wonder whether I'll be able to give up. I fly
to Connecticut about once a month to see Mike. The day
before, I shave my legs, slather my body in moisturizer, and
dream about meeting him at the airport. In my fantasies, our
eyes meet, we rush into each other's arms and lock lips in a
passionate kiss. The day of my trip I shower, make sure my
legs are still smooth, put on a short skirt or something else I
know Mike favors, apply lipstick, and spray perfume in places
that count. While I'm getting ready, I listen to loud rock and
roll, breaking out into an occasional dance. Often the songs
are about betrayal or hearts rent asunder, music I can only
appreciate when I am hours rather than weeks away from
seeing Mike.

The flight always seems unbearably long, and when I dis-
embark, I anxiously search the crowd for his dark head, which
stands out because he is quite tall. When I spot him, I can't
catch my breath for a moment. Instead of running, we walk
quickly toward each other. Sometimes I am struck with a
sudden bout of shyness and cannot look into his eyes; I burrow into his arms instead. It's never like the rapturous meeting
I imagined, but I don't care. My fantasies are replaced with
the equally satisfying feeling of having his solid presence beside me, Mike with me in flesh and blood, his arm resting
easily on my shoulder.

That's another reason I do not mind what many would
call "contrived" romance. It usually does not fluster me if
things do not progress exactly as planned; I adjust without
realizing it. Then again, events often unfold pretty much the

way I envisioned, the result, I think, of how readily I assume
whatever romantic role I cast for myself. The two men whom
I've loved deeply do the same. My first boyfriend used to tell
me stories while we made love. I was lying on some sun-
drenched beach and a strange man began to caress me; I was
a queen and he was my servant. I can't remember most of the
stories he told; I only remember that I was carried away by
them, that if something he said suddenly sounded absurd or
funny, I did not dwell on it. Mike sometimes lights candles
in the bedroom; he puts on a Chet Baker tape that he knows
makes me swoon. I seduce him with lingerie I ordered from,
yes, Victoria's Secret. I bought him an erotic novel, which
we read to each other in bed while lightly, even absently,
stroking each other's bodies. Eventually, the sensuous prose
drives us together. The fact that we both could have predicted
the passion that the music, the novel, the candlelight provoke
does not diminish the wonder of it.

Not all of my romantic setups are designed for immediate
sexual gratification, though they often are extended preludes
to lovemaking. Vacations fall into this category. I think of the
cross-country ski trip Mike and I took one New Year's holiday. We stayed at a bed-and-breakfast and in four days developed a sexy but relaxing routine. We woke around 9 a.m. and
made love, then had breakfast in a dining room with soaring
windows that overlooked wild, wintery Lake Superior. Then
we skiied until our muscles ached, came home, peeled off our
damp clothes, and did it again. We took a hot shower, had
dinner at a low-key restaurant or fixed a frozen pizza, drank
beer, played cards, and if we still had the energy. . . .

When I am with Mike, I try to make as many evenings as
possible "special," or romantic. Not that I cook all day—I
don't have the time or the talent. It means Mike and I go out
to dinner, or I cook one of my three standard pasta dishes
and we eat by candlelight. I also celebrate most any holiday
I can, Hallmark-created or not. I can think of two friends

who boast that they never do anything obviously romantic
with their boyfriends on Valentine's Day. It's too commercial, they complain. Expectations are too high. My response? A blinding blizzard could not keep me from
romance on Valentine's Day.

The worst blizzard in Chicago in recent memory was on
Valentine's Day 1990. It usually takes me twenty minutes to
drive home from work; that day it took three white-knuckled
hours to bring in my boat of car, a 1976 Cordoba. Mike and
I had planned to have dinner at the Como Inn, an ornate,
unabashedly romantic Neapolitan restaurant. I know some
people who would go here as a joke on Valentine's Day and
laugh all the way through the meal. Ha, ha, ha, isn't this
corny? But Mike and I did not intend to dine with our tongues
in cheek; this wasn't the David Letterman show. By the time
I got home at 8:15, I was tired and the thought of getting
back into the car was daunting, but neither of us wanted to
forgo the evening we had planned. So I took a quick shower
and shoved off in the Cordoba. By the time I arrived, the
restaurant was nearly empty. Few were so stupid as to venture
out this night. When I walked through the door, I immediately saw Mike sitting at the bar. He was wearing a white
shirt, nice tie, and fine dark pants; he knows how to dress for
a special occasion. He was accepting the attentions of a lonely
woman, which did not bother me a bit. Eyes do not lie; as
soon as Mike's caught mine, I felt desired.

The restaurant is the kind where couples get their own
small alcoves, and as we slid into ours, we could not help
noticing the collective sigh of the serving staff. We had bol-
lixed their chance to go home early. On an objective level,
things did not get much better from there. The chef had
stopped preparing several of the entrees we wanted, and everyone seemed to be hurrying us along. Then, when we were
ready to go, the Cordoba would not start. I had planned to

go back to Mike's anyway, so we left my car in the snowy parking lot and glided home in his.

I have fond memories of that night. It was Valentine's Day, and Mike and I willed our romantic evening into being. We went the extra mile for each other.

Romance II

CARROLL STONER

I crave romance about as much as I am suspicious of it.

First the craving. My desire for romance hasn't changed much over the years, although I have. I still have the fantasy of being kissed, passionately, on a beach in Mexico when it is winter up north where I live. The reality of my life makes that difficult. My husband sunburns easily. He grew up in a summer community and he hates the messiness of sand. He does not love Mexico as I do. If there were an island run by German engineers, we would go there—although he understands that tropical climates mean that his idealized, perfectly run island kingdom will never exist, that even Middle Europeans lose their by-the-rules efficiency in the constant sunshine. Most of all, though, the idea of making love on a beach is preposterous, as out of the question as necking in the middle of Marshall Field's at high noon. If we are all alone in our car and I lean over to kiss him, he looks both ways in a broadly comedic way, as if he were one of the Marx Brothers and

afraid of being caught doing something embarrassing, which
is what he thinks of public displays of affection.

I want candlelit dinners for two, where we look deep into
each other's eyes as proof that we love each other after all
these years and can still laugh and be interested by each other's fresh ideas and original mind. He likes that, too, and once
in a while we go to an Italian or French or contemporary
American place that specializes in trendy food and terrific atmosphere. But mostly we stay home or take one or more of
our children to storefront ethnic restaurants.

I love sunsets in places like Mexico, where it's a special
time of day, awaited eagerly and greeted by crowds in a daily
ritual planned around watching something beautiful. We once
had an apartment that faced east and had views of each day's
sunrise. Some back windows—one overlooking a fire escape,
the other in the laundry room—faced west, so we had sunsets,
too, although we never watched them, which says something
both about building construction in the 1920s and about the
perfectionism of romance. A sunset isn't the same when it's
viewed across a Maytag.

There is no doubt that one component of romance's appeal
is its scarcity, probably because humans disdain anything they
can too easily get. When I was young, I didn't want any of
the men who wanted me, which was probably my way of
avoiding entanglement. By the time I married (the real time),
at twenty-nine, I was the woman I wanted to become and he
liked who I was. By that time, also, I had cast aside some
illusions about true love and romance and about myself. At
almost thirty and close to forty, we were ready to commit to
taking care of each other, because we'd finally learned to take
care of ourselves. We were no longer looking for perfection in
a mate, although we both admit to being smitten the first
evening we met (at a party) and spent the first years of our
marriage thinking we were the perfect couple, with some kind
of magical bond between us. It was a second marriage and we

needed romance. We went out of our way to be romantic for
years, often in a self-conscious, this-marriage-is-going-to-work
manner. He always picked me up from work so that we could
be together for the time it took to get from the newspaper
where I worked to our house ten blocks away. I fixed the
foods he loved—all the time. We often ate late, just the two
of us, with candlelight.

I discovered then how much we both love spontaneous
and romantic gestures, although I also sometimes find them
embarrassing. An old boyfriend used to send armloads of
flowers, which never helped his position in my life, since I
simply didn't like him that much. Now, when my husband
sends me flowers, I love it. Several times he has come home
with not one but two boxes of garden flowers, so that I could
arrange them in the natural style I like. I was touched by that
because it showed he knew what I was thinking about. I
would not have been nearly as thrilled by long-stemmed roses,
which I think are overpriced for such predictable flowers. He
knows that I prefer bunches of French lilacs or flowering
branches or wildflowers. I'm not acquisitive enough to have
"trained" him, women's shorthand for telling a man, again and
again, what is important to them. In fact, I get distinctly
uncomfortable when I think he has spent too much, which
surely gives him a mixed message—that he should buy me
beautiful things, but never spend more than my undefined,
unspoken comfort level allows me to accept.

I think that love is frightening and powerful and I believe
we create romance to make it less so. What we choose to
romanticize is revealing about us. We idealize subjects that
seduce as well as repel us, that frighten us as well as attract
us because of their inherent power. Like love. (And sex and
lust.) Love is powerful. Irrational. Kingdoms have been won
and lost over it. Men and women still do incredibly wonderful
or terrible things in its name. I have watched intelligent
friends do stupid things in the name of love, as if they have

suddenly taken leave of their senses. Romance is an especially
strong component of the female psyche, revealing a strong
need to idealize things. Like love. (And sex and lust.)

Years ago I read something by anthropologist Margaret
Mead about romantic love. I found it in a book of her columns, written in response to a question about whether romantic love and marriage could mix. It ran in *Redbook* in 1965,
when I was twenty-two, and it still impresses me with its
wisdom and clarity. Among other things, she wrote:

> Society has domesticated what is essentially a very antiso-
> cial idea. For what the world needs is not romantic lovers
> who are sufficient unto themselves, but husbands and
> wives who live in communities, relate to other people,
> carry on useful work and willingly give time and attention
> to their children.
>
> The individual who is immersed in extreme romantic
> love is obsessed by the beloved person, desperately un-
> happy in his or her absence and wholly unconcerned with
> the activities of everyday life. It is a state of mind that
> requires a vast overestimation of the loved one, who is
> visualized as flawless and incomparable.

That sense of perfection, of the glory of having found each
other, was what my husband and I felt in the throes of romantic love, and I sometimes mourn its demise.

Clearly, with her multiple unions, Mead never mastered
marriage, unless serial marriages count (maybe romantics keep
getting divorced and remarried so that they can be in a constant state of romantic love). Studying freer societies could
have made the limits of traditional Western marriage intoler-
able. I read that she did all her own housework and was forced
by one of her husbands to do it out of his sight, since he
couldn't stand to see her performing demeaning domestic
tasks. That says more about her willingness to compromise

than anything I've read about her. Don't tell me she didn't look for romantic love, even though she understood its limitations.

It is clear that submissiveness, compromise, and constant concession make women deeply angry. It also seems obvious that a big part of romance is built around the idea of having a man take care of us, and that this is something of a one-way street. He invites *me* out to dinner. He sends *me* flowers. He buys *me* gifts. In reality, I don't reciprocate much, although I should, since I know that my husband is also romantic. Like it or not, my notions of romance clearly express that old need to be taken care of.

At the same time, my ambivalence is rooted in suspicion, grounded in the idea that much of what we call romance is fakery salted with helplessness to make us feel better about . . . something we don't really like. Example: Nancy Reagan might have been a less angry woman if she hadn't forced herself to sit and look up at her husband at every public appearance in that rapt way that gave onlookers false hopes for romantic devotion and that must have literally given her a pain in the neck. In reality their marriage sounds almost remarkably devoid of emotional intensity or shared reflection.

Do I, fast approaching fifty, still need romance?

In exactly the way Margaret Mead described romantic love, when we first married my husband and I felt that together we became a complete human being, while apart we were incomplete. We didn't just talk, we devoured each other's thoughts, feelings, attitudes. We found them exciting, wondrous. We were in love and, yes, we idealized each other. I hate the idea that when romantic love dies, a fuller, more mature love replaces it, which sounds like a bad bargain and a disingenuous rationalization to boot.

My husband on romance, off the top of his head: "Romance to me is intense intimacy, sometimes deliberate, sometimes spontaneous. The key is the intensity of feeling. I don't always understand what generates those feelings, in an intellectual sense, but when I feel romantic I want to reach out and make the feeling so apparent that it generates the same feeling in you." (No wonder I love him.)

We've had many such shared moments. And then, a few years ago we discovered that they were happening less and less often. For some deeply unacknowledged reasons, we had grown angry with each other. We ignored these feelings, believing it was another tired inevitability of a long-term marriage. Even though we knew we needed romance and that it grows out of time alone and shared thoughts and feelings, we did nothing.

For years, when things were better, we had had a sacrosanct Wednesday-night date, when we went out alone and spent time together. What we did wasn't important. Sometimes we went to the theater or to a restaurant or movie. Occasionally we went to a blues or jazz club. And once or twice we went somewhere and argued all night. Nevertheless, this time alone fueled our marriage.

Recently, after a couple of difficult years, we fell in love again. I had spent a few weeks with our family in a country cottage while he continued to work in the city. When we got back together, that old feeling was back. Intellectually, I know why it happened. With the help of marriage counseling we were seeing new facets of each other and had begun to acknowledge our anger and its causes. I had joined a women's group and was feeling nourished by it. And absence had made our hearts softer. But being back "in love" was more feeling than anything rational. We nursed it along and it lasted awhile and during that time it felt like another honeymoon. We were especially thoughtful of each other and that fed something deep within us that needed to be cherished. It was a reminder of how marriage can be.

As recently as three days ago we resolved, again, to find time for each other, and yesterday we managed an afternoon alone. We wandered through an art museum, looking at his favorite category of art, photography, as well as mine, furniture and art objects—making sure we saw both and not just one. We ended our visit on neutral ground, with some paintings we both admire. We didn't plan our route, we just gravitated to the galleries we each know the other likes. We were late getting started and it was four by the time we left the museum, so our idea of a romantic lunch fell in the middle of that short time when it is too late for an elegant lunch and too early for dinner. (A friend later reminded me that expensive hotels always have elegant restaurants for off-hours occasions, something I find worth noting.) Then, too, we had to be home in time to take our daughter to swimming practice at six.

We ended up eating slices of pizza in the car in front of our favorite Italian bakery and delicatessen, where we stocked up on crusty Italian bread and some other treats. But candlelight must have ignited somewhere, because that night, after our daughter had finally finished a school project and was safely in bed, we went to our own bed and ate grilled slices of the Italian bread spread with ripe St. André cheese and draped with slices of rosy prosciutto. We talked some more and then we brushed the crumbs out of bed.

It was one of those incredibly intimate, delicate moments that are as fragile and fleeting as a sunset. We didn't have to open a bottle of wine or light candles. There was no lace or flowers. But it was gentle and loving and one of those moments that define romance for us.

ℒosing 𝒞ontrol

JANICE SOMERVILLE

June

I sipped my beer at the restaurant across from his apartment. I checked my watch. I walked outside into the stifling heat, in case he happened to drive by. I checked my watch. I went back into the bar and picked up a newspaper. I put it down and went to the phone. No answer.

Where was he? My heart raced, I couldn't sit still. I checked my watch. I took a deep breath and tried to calm down to keep myself from shaking the waiter and every customer there, demanding an answer.

I had never been one to wait by the phone. And I had certainly never staked out a man's home before. But I didn't care. I wanted no part of rational thought or common sense. I had leaped off the edge, but I hadn't fallen; I was soaring. And like the downhill racer who knows that self-doubt is deadly, I believed if I ever doubted my instincts I would lose my balance and crash.

My instincts told me not to believe or even listen to his occasional warnings that his future probably didn't include marriage or me—he wanted to keep himself open to all of life's possibilities, including, of course, other women. If I didn't trust these instincts, I believed, I would recklessly give him an ultimatum. And that would only drive him away.

I wanted only to immerse myself in him. Finally, I had

fallen in love with a man I liked, respected, and admired. And I lusted after him with the most primal urges I had ever felt. Incredibly, he returned my ardor with equal intensity. If I held myself in check, or waited for a more stable relationship, I would always know that I had turned my back on the greatest chance I had ever had to indulge in all-encompassing, intoxicating lust or love, or whatever it was; I didn't particularly care.

I craved his company, I craved his body, but most of all, I craved the intense feelings that swept everything else aside. And so I was hurtling through space, embracing all of it, even the agonizing moments, like the hot summer nights I spent keeping a secret vigil outside his apartment.

And eventually, anyway, he would answer the phone. "Hello," he said finally, that night in June.

Relief surging through my body, I took a deep breath and said casually, "Hi, what are you doing?"

"Not much. I just got in from the bookstore."

"Did you buy anything?" I asked.

"The Hemingway book. There's a part I'd really like to read to you. Can you come over?"

"Actually, I was in the neighborhood, so I stopped for a drink, in case you came home soon. I'm across the street."

When I reached his third-floor, un-air-conditioned studio, he wore, as usual that summer, only his shorts. His hair was slightly tousled, and his skin shone from a shower. He smiled and hugged me hard.

We made love and I slept soundly all night.

July

The summer grew hotter, becoming one long, record-breaking heat wave. The grass in Lincoln Park turned yellow, and spring-fed Lake Michigan felt like stale bathwater. Even with air-conditioning, most of my friends said it was too hot to make love. We couldn't stop.

I had a roommate and a smaller bed, so we were rarely at my apartment. Instead, we spent hour after hour in his tiny studio, which had room for only a bed and his desk and a portable fan. We spent nearly all of our time on the bed. We watched rented movies, paid our bills, made our phone calls, read to each other, and ate there, primarily Jell-O squares, fruit juice, and shakes made with fresh strawberries because it was too hot to cook. We also had long talks on his bed, although I recall little of what we said, only the soothing cadences of his voice, full of honesty, tenderness, and passion.

Sometimes I would recall bits of stories and movies about other lovers, but I pushed them out of my mind, because I didn't want to be reminded that anyone else had ever experienced such a love affair, or that the things we said and did might sound trite by comparison. Nor did I want to recall that so many tales, like *9½ Weeks* or *Anna Karenina*, ended badly. Above all, I didn't want to remember that such a feeling couldn't last, or that if it did, it would probably destroy us.

He was serious and quiet, the first quiet man I had ever dated. I was usually attracted to cynics and wits and extroverts, men who loved late-night conversation at smoky neighborhood bars. But I discovered that summer that he was not always quiet; it was just that he shared his thoughts with only the few people he believed would appreciate them. And I discovered that he was not always serious, that he had a gentle but ironic sense of humor, and that he could be as irreverent as intense.

And I discovered his body, his strong hands, and his gentle touch. I wanted only to lie next to him and trace my hands over his taut muscles. He had the body of an athlete, but not the overdeveloped muscles of the serious competitor, and he moved with a sensual grace. His eyes reflected feelings that he did not always tell me.

I couldn't sit still. I couldn't concentrate at work. I couldn't share our time with anyone. I recalled my parents' tenets of a happy marriage: "A healthy relationship needs balance. Never neglect your friends, and don't try to do everything together. Have hobbies of your own."

I waved such words aside, although I believed in them. That summer, there was no room for anything but us.

August

Toward the end of the month, we could no longer stand the heat, and we fled his apartment. But the city's beachfront offered no relief, none of the comfort it gave in other summers.

The air was thick, and the water felt almost gelatinous as we waded along the shore to escape the burning sand. A hot wind blew in from the city, bringing all its soot and grime and dirt. Bits of candy wrappers and cigarette butts spun into the air, swirling around our faces. I wistfully recalled spring days with clear blue skies and fresh breezes and frigid winter days when the ice glistened on the lake and trees. We held hands, though it was so hot that even that small contact was nearly unbearable.

The grass behind us had turned brown and even the oaks were drooping. I couldn't remember when it had last rained. But the sky was darkening, turning an apocalyptic green. Instead of running for cover, however, we grinned with anticipation. A drop fell on my face. Several more followed, then torrents. We shouted and let go of hands to hold them up to the sky, wanting to feel every drop. We were drenched in seconds, and the rain pounded our faces, but we couldn't leave. Then, as quickly as it had started, the rain stopped, and we slowly walked home.

The summer dragged on, with no more storms, and now we always noticed the heat. We began escaping to the dark coolness of movie theaters and restaurants, and he began to ask me questions like "Where do you usually meet men?"

He worried that his life was in a rut, and he told me that he wanted to meet more people.

Our affair grew more lopsided than ever, and I began to think about ending it. But our lovemaking had a sharper edge that thrilled me, as we began to sense that we did not have much time left together. And when it was over, and we were apart for another day, sometimes two or three now, my fears and longing for him intensified. Even if I wanted to stop, to stop schussing down the mountain, I couldn't safely turn at such a high speed. I'd have to wait until the slope leveled out.

September

We spent less and less time together, and I began to care less and less about everything that had ever mattered to me. Finally, I felt so emotionally drained that I managed to tell him, "I can't do this anymore." A week later he told me he had met someone else. He also said that he didn't want to give me up, and several of the other well-meaning but devastating platitudes that people say when they are moving on without you.

I went for a walk later that night. The weather, sunny and warm hours before, had turned cold and damp. Suddenly it was fall. The summer and its unfathomable heat were just figures for the record books. I shivered with the unfamiliar cold, and I ached, not just for him, for his voice and his touch, but for the intensity of the moments we had shared, and for the passing of a time in my life when I would embrace such a risk.

I knew that I would never forget what it feels like to crash, and while I believed that the memories were worth the pain, that they would not make me bitter, I also knew that they would haunt me. I would become careful. A sharp wind whipped around me, and I pulled my jacket tighter around my shoulders.

The Car

My trip to work takes nearly an hour down winding exurban
roads clogged with panel trucks, station wagons, and cars with
rear-window decals announcing the colleges their owners' children have chosen. Traffic copters barely take notice of commuters like us, though we number in the millions. Spilling
from our split ranches and center-hall colonials, we pour out
the driveways and into the river of cars cutting through old
country towns and subdivision suburbs. Long commutes
down roads designed for another century are the rule. I spend
so much time in my car that it is a second home, littered, like
my house, with books and food and laundry.

Some commuters eat breakfast in the car—one double
decaf with milk and sugar, one scone for me—some put on
their makeup, some attend to the final details of personal
grooming. Once I watched a balding man with a ponytail,
wearing what looked like an Italian suit, picking his nose rumi-
natively as his Lexus idled at the light. On the way into the
office each morning, I run my fingers through my wet hair to
dry it and fluff it up. On the way back at night, when I think
no one can see me, I wriggle out of my thigh-high stockings,
one leg per red light, and drive home barefoot. Despite tapes
of mysteries and *Morning Edition*, it is a boring commute.
When I can, I watch the drivers around me. We all do, check-

ing out each other's faces in our rear-views, looking sidelong at each other at the red lights.

Our quick glances are not furtive, just careful: Lights change, cars move, and we have to keep our eyes on the traffic. Subway commuters are the ones who must be furtive, sneaking glances as quickly and thoroughly as they can without engaging a return look. One of the pleasures of auto-voyeurism is that it is discreet and remote. On the train to town, I cannot avoid my seatmate. I smell his aftershave. We jostle subtly for a larger slice of the seat. On a train, if you want, you can talk. And sometimes, if you don't want to talk, you can't avoid it. If you get caught peeking at your neighbor, it invites conversation, not all of it nice. In my car, on the other hand, I can size up my fellow travelers more openly. I may imagine whatever I want about them and, even if they can read my thoughts, there is nothing they can do about it. Two windows and two reassuring doors separate commuters and their imaginations from one another.

Only once did I want to break those barriers. A few weeks ago, on one of those wonderfully sunny, sky-blue December mornings we get around here, I looked in my rear-view mirror to see an Isuzu truck almost balanced on my tailpipe. The driver was my kind of handsome, with a face that was lived-in rather than pretty. Made of angles and planes weathered by time, his was a face a sculptor could do something with. I couldn't see his eyes at that distance, but his granny glasses made him look intelligent. (Some women are drawn to cleft chins or hairy chests. I am a sucker for a man in gold-rimmed glasses. I married one.) The driver's cheekbones were strong, his chin square, his mouth wide, but not so wide that he looked like a jack-o'-lantern. He seemed about thirty. I thought he might be smiling at me. I smiled at his reflection in my mirror.

My first thought wasn't so much a thought as a perception of energy, the kind of lift I used to get from the Supremes.

Smiling at him and feeling the sense of possibility flood through me felt as good as when I was an eleventh-grader driving home from my best friend's house singing whatever Motown had at the top of the charts. I considered dropping back, changing lanes, and letting him pull up alongside me so that I could look and smile again. Maybe he would look and smile back.

But what would happen next? Would we pull over to the curb and talk? Exchange phone numbers? And then what? That happened to me once on the way to work, when a tall thin man in cowboy boots, Levis, and an ersatz Stetson waited at the bus next to me. I was aware of him, attracted to him, and, to cover my self-consciousness, I pulled out my book when we boarded the crowded bus, and tried to read standing up as we lurched toward the Loop. He got off the bus with me, and said, "I want to know what kind of girl can read a book on the bus." He worked in my building, he said. "Can I call you later?" he asked. I gave him my number and we headed for our different elevator banks. The phone rang within the hour. The resulting affair turned out badly because I wanted to fall in love and he didn't. I picked him for the worst of reasons—I was at loose ends. But my folly shouldn't turn anyone off from a chance encounter. I also met my husband through a chance encounter. In these matters, timing is everything. Not only was he a good man, he wanted a family. So did I. We were bursting with the need to love someone. We wanted to settle down.

Settled, married, and with a family, I *still* wished I could breach the walls and talk to the man in the Isuzu on a car phone, except that I didn't have one and, judging by the rust on the truck, neither did he. Nor do I know how to find a car phone number. Stymied, with no way to attract his attention and not cause an accident and without the courage to act even if I'd had the means, I retreated to fantasy. When we met, what would I say? The obvious sounded ludicrous—"I have a husband and two children, but it made me feel good to look at you so I wanted to stop and say hello." Anything I said would be embarrassing. In a flirtation, the margin for misunderstanding is so thin. It is very easy to send the wrong signals.

What if it got serious? And what was the point otherwise? The beauty of fantasy is that you don't have to answer the questions. In your imagination, there's no need to walk the fine line between friendship, which is rooted in shared skills and shared ideas, and flirtation, which concentrates on sex and romance. Besides, I am at a stage of my life where flirtation is unbecoming, unnecessary, and unwelcome. I have outlived its usefulness. Flirting is girlish, and I am a woman. Past a certain age (which I have passed), it is as difficult to flirt grace-fully as it is to look good in a short skirt. Flirting is best learned in grade school, refined in high school, polished in college, and jettisoned before the age of thirty.

During my aching, awkward adolescence, nothing pre-pared me for courtship, just for friendship, and in the long run friendships are what count, not flirtations. But once in a while, like that morning on the road, I miss the electric undercurrent, the sexual alertness, the spice of possibility, that runs through flirtations.

I stopped trying to imagine myself talking to him in a gallery (I met someone there once, too), dropped my line of thinking, and turned the radio to an oldies station. Loving the sunny morning and the idea of a handsome man in the car behind me, I began to sing along. I thought about the benefits of being single and unattached—walking into a room filled with people and possibility, checking out the crowd to see who was there, sometimes singling out one man, then maneuvering around the room to be near him so that I could measure the resonance of his voice, the sense of his words. Had that once been me? While I was daydreaming and not paying much attention to anything besides how good I felt, he changed lanes and shot ahead. I tried to catch up.

No matter how fast I drove and how often I changed lanes, I wasn't able to pull alongside the Isuzu until I was near the turnoff for my office. Before I turned, I took a good look at him. He was my age, give or take, and still looked rough-hewn and craggy, though his neck sagged like mine. He started to turn my way. I looked up at the light. It turned. I swung left into the parking lot and he pulled ahead. I wished he could have known he was the object of my fantasy and thought it might have made him feel at least a little bit as good as I felt.

Postscript. The man in the Isuzu reads this book. He sees this essay. He calls me up. I ask him who he is and he says, "I am the rest of your life."

LETTING GO

Sexy

CARROLL STONER

I haven't known many men or women I considered sexy. I believe this is because for years, my definition was slightly off, colored by adolescent fantasies. More to the point, every subject related to sexuality is more instinctive than intellectual, and I didn't allow my antennae to work.

Actually, I think I'm put off by displays of blatant sexuality. I don't think I'm alone. Isn't there something odd, suspicious, even a little embarrassing about men and women who parade their sexuality? Think of Elvis Presley, the world's best parody of male sexiness. Or about the vulnerable, sexual image projected by Marilyn Monroe, an abandoned and abused child who never could get enough male approval. On the other hand, I recently met a woman who says she spotted her husband because he was the sexiest boy in second grade. I think that's amazing. That he was. And that she recognized it.

Where I grew up, thinking of oneself as sexy would have required beating major, albeit invisible odds, or so I thought when I was young. In my predominantly Lutheran, middle-class Minnesota small-town-turned-suburb, being blond and slim seemed more like being colorless and flat-chested. And although cool Scandinavians are by some strange, twisted reasoning considered hot-blooded, I can't think of any girl in town who was considered sexy, not even Sharon Carlson, who, according to my boyfriend and his friend, didn't have a stitch on under her robe when we all stopped by one afternoon to visit.

Sharon Carlson? Naked under her robe? How could they tell? And why did they care? Now, I recognize boys' sexual curiosity and wish girls felt free to express more of it, but then I had no idea. I remember this small, surprising peek into the minds of these sixteen-year-old boys as one of the first glimpses I got into the world of men and sex, which at the time seemed exotic and appealing and scary—and sometimes still does.

Somewhere in my mind I had a vision of what was sexy: A moody, dark, slightly menacing quality is as close as I can come to defining it. To be sexy was to be complicated, whereas the popular personality of the moment was open, fun-loving, a girl who smiled a lot. "Peppy" was actually a word we used to describe something we liked in each other.

But blond and Minnesotan or no, there was some rebellious, libidinous self-image forming inside me somewhere, because at sixteen I had a short, red, low-cut formal, as we called them, made for the prom. I wore it with long, dangling rhinestone earrings (I think I got the idea from the Miss America pageant), dyed-to-match high heels, and short red kid gloves. To provide some perspective, this was in the era of floor-length pastels, long white gloves, and flat shoes worn to make your date seem taller. A year later, when we all wore our formals to sing in the spring choir concert, a freshman told me I looked "just like a nightclub singer," and I remember feeling happy that he got the message that I was different, unconventional. Good. Maybe I was more chanteuse than Future Homemaker of America.

I never told my mother about the remark, since I was in that predictable teenage hiatus from speaking to her much at all. I think it would have pleased her, since she had groomed her three daughters to "be different" and "stand out from the crowd." She must have devoted some serious thought to those intentions because she often went off on carefully crafted tangents about how important it was to live life for yourself, rather than for the approval of others. I was not at all sure she was right, but in some measure I think her message stuck.

My mother. Although she died when I was twenty-one, she still lives in my head and is my measure of the real (as opposed to the conventional) notions of good and bad, right and wrong, rational and too-dumb-to-be-believed. She was savvy, wise, nobody's fool. On the other hand, it's impossible for me to know what kind of woman she was in private, since all our adult conversations died with her. I can guess that she was passionate, because she had strong convictions about everything in a quiet, controlled, Protestant sort of way.

After her death, I complained to her best friend that I'd ne___ witnessed any affection between my parents. Had they l_____ ___? And Kay, a salty, straightforward woman, t_____ __ain terms that my mother and father had _____ __riage. Didn't I remember how my mother _____ __d fixed her hair every afternoon before my _____ __om work? But the evidence of sexuality I _____ outward, more physical, like when I'd seen __ father back her mother into a corner of their _____ __oth palms against the wall at the level of his _____ __s, and give her a long, lingering kiss. Patty _____ __p, and shrugged as if to say, "Oh them," while _____ __bstruck, in the doorway and stared. But maybe _____ __ctation of passion isn't so great either, now that _____ __, since Patty admitted many years later that she'd div_____ __er first husband and married his best friend because he gave her what she described as "bells and banjos." And then she left this man who had helped her raise a bunch of kids, for a third husband who, I assume, appealed to her even more.

Is Patty sexy? I think she might be, although I'm not sure
of my perceptions about women, especially those I knew as
children.

Sexy men are easier to spot, if only because of the physical
reaction they inspire. I've been involved with only three men
I thought from the moment I met them were incredibly sexy,
and involvement with one was limited to elaborate fantasies
built around a single but memorable kiss after I'd let him copy
my algebra answers when I was a high school freshman and
he was a junior. I think he kissed me out of gratitude. It was
also to let me know he was in charge, even if he wasn't good
at math. After that one kiss, he flirted with me enough to
keep my innocent freshman heart pumping. The fantasies I
had about him had little to do with sex but a lot to do with
romance and consisted of long, lingering kisses and of gazing
deep into each other's eyes in surroundings that were vague,
but sort of foggy and warm—London in August? This boy
was surely aware of my adulation, since I spent all of algebra
class looking at him, imagining what kissing him again would
be like. I'm not sure, but I think that if I ran into him today
I'd be thrown into a state of sexual confusion. More than
anyone I've met since growing up, I think this boy could have
made me feel loved, because at fourteen I felt so totally unlov-
able and because he had such a strong personality. A sexual
relationship, of course, would have been out of the question,
since I was intent on being a good girl. He, on the other hand,
was dangerous, the first of many men I liked who projected
controlled menace. He was sexy.

The next time I was overwhelmed by lust at first sight, I
was in my early twenties, and I remember feeling absolutely
frantic to make love to the man who caused this sexual frisson.
Keeping him at bay for the required several dates before I
"gave in" and we made love was difficult, but I sensed that
once we started, we would never do anything else—and then
there was the "will he love me in the morning?" question. I

now wish I hadn't had to rationalize being in love with him after we started sleeping together, since my heart still bears the scars. What we had was great, but I don't think it had a thing to do with love.

What I know now that I didn't recognize then is that both of these boy-men shared qualities that once fascinated me: Narcissistic and unloving, they were dark, with a good amount of controlled danger to their personalities.

My oldest friend recalls that as a girl I went for dangerous boys, and they for me, which I now believe expressed a deep yearning not to have to be so relentlessly cheerful. Dangerous boys liked me because I was a good girl, straight as an arrow, a cheerleader who liked to step out on the wild side. Most of them had early bloomer written all over them, which is dangerous for men. Boys who get lots of early sexual approval from women often seem emotionally retarded when they grow up, maybe because they don't have to work at development and never do mature.

In the long run the qualities that inspired early sexual fantasy were not much to build a life on. Feeling out of control has never been a harbinger for me of anything good to come in a relationship. Perhaps, because of some difficult family circumstances involving a schizophrenic half-brother, I seldom felt safe enough as a young woman to intentionally lose control. Even as a little girl, I struggled to be cheerful and optimistic and in control. It took me years to see that one could be all of those things as well as sensual.

By college I had recognized that almost no men express sexuality as openly as those high school bad boys had. For a few years in my twenties I mistakenly thought power and success made men sexy, which was pure projection, since I wanted to be powerful and successful myself. About then I figured out what that sense of controlled danger had meant to me: Somehow, it put them in charge. I saw those bad boys as capable of taking charge of my pleasure, since I was so

fearful of it myself. Again, the issue of control that has been
so central to my life.

Over the years I've learned to recognize a sexually confident man when I meet one, and I still have a private scorecard
of the men I find sexually attractive. I have had three sexy
bosses over the years, and one who was overtly sexual. He
told bawdy jokes at the drop of a hat and he was decidedly
unsexy. It is not sexy to be too obviously sexual.

Maybe it's age, but my antennae not only work now, they
home in on subtleties. I watch men with women. At parties,
I watch them dance. If I see a couple who move well together,
and if they do a very small amount of sexual acting out—a
leg rubbing, a hand moving on an arm, a palm firmly planted
on the lower back, if there's the sense that they're engaged
with each other, then I believe they have a good, mutually
satisfying sex life, which is what sexuality is all about. I recently watched a man, a nervous and jumpy guy who happens
not to be very attractive but who is married to an elegant
woman, and he was running his hand down his wife's behind
and holding her upper arm and caressing her in other, half-
conscious ways, and I realized that he is a sexual man. Sexy?
Not to me. But sexual? You bet.

Sexuality is about pleasure and passion and satisfaction and
the confidence to lose control, and a great part of humanity
knows about it. Sexiness is alluring and seductive, image and
perception. It is powerful and scary because it invites sexual
response, and because it is so rare.

Call it confidence or wisdom or simply age and experience.
I know that good sex and being sexy or sexual or both don't
always work together. Looking back, I think that separating
some Hollywood version of sexuality from my own feelings
about it was important, and that the differences between sexiness and sexuality are elusive. I got over the confusion in
time to marry someone who is both sexy and deeply sexual
without being frightening. And although the dynamic of our

marriage is a too-frequent struggle for power and control, the intimate part of our relationship has never been a source of worry.

My husband has instant antennae for sexiness. Years ago, when I told him about a political reporter who had been having an affair with a politician and who made the fatal mistake of taking a mink coat from the guy and who'd been fired because of it, he knew who I was talking about even though he'd never met her. "She has long dark hair, an incredibly sexy walk and broad shoulders, is about five-five and looks like she has a Southern accent," he said with complete certainty. I was dumbstruck. All this from seeing her coming and going at the newspaper where I also worked. Everyone knew she was sexy, including the man who assigned her to cover politics and who later feigned shock over her dalliance. She was set apart by her overt sensuality, and I remember feeling a little childish in her company even though we were approximately the same age. Like Debbie Reynolds meeting Ava Gardner. I used to watch her cross the newsroom, and watch every man in the place stop working to look up and follow her progress. It was an amazing sight. She did something between a sashay and an amble, the most sensuous walk I've ever seen.

I recently met a couple who I guessed were well matched and happily married. I met him ten minutes before I met his wife, and while we were waiting for her to join us, I asked him about his job and his life. He leaned against the sprawling log cabin they had built together on the shores of Lake Tahoe, a slim, intense, brown-haired man of no particular beauty. While we were talking, I realized he was an incredibly sexy man of the type I had once craved. He had a masterful sense of control about him. Not surprisingly, he is a card dealer at one of the most elegant, high-stakes casinos in Nevada. Later, during a leisurely, wine-filled lunch overlooking the lake, his wife told our mutual friend and me that she had been in love with him since he was in second grade and she was in first, when she thought he was the sexiest boy alive. They started going steady at fourteen and have been married for over twenty-five years, and it was obvious that they are still attracted to each other. I think they are lucky.

Having recently lost some weight, I am considering buying a black lace bustier to wear for the holidays. I'm still trying to define what being sexy might mean for me. Wearing black lace in public is a tempting idea, one that looks fairly adventurous and risky to a married woman approaching fifty. I haven't made up my mind about it.

But women who have invented themselves in the first place know how to take risks. And I think that matters of taste aside, when I got that red dress, I took the first innocent step toward being the woman I wanted to be, who was both sexy and sexual. Even before I knew how different sexiness and sexuality are, I wanted both. I recognize that my mother had the two qualities and that she knew it and wanted the same for me. I wish I could ask her opinion on the black lace bustier. Maybe, like the red dress I could be excused for when I was sixteen, it's too obvious. She would be eighty-three if she had lived, but I think she'd laugh.

Just Looking

JANICE SOMERVILLE

"Your problem is that you're looking too hard. I wasn't looking at all when I met Jim," said my friend, with the smug and self-congratulatory tone of a woman who had found the right man. "I couldn't have cared less whether I met anyone or not. I was having too much fun just dating and working." She must be right, I thought, forgetting her previous, unfaithful boyfriends and the nights she spent wailing that she would never get married.

The answer to the dilemma was radiantly clear. I would let men know that, frankly, I was happy with my life, and that I didn't care whether I found my Heathcliff or not. Fervently, I practiced not looking. I didn't look at bars or restaurants or parties. I didn't look on buses. Instead, I focused on the people I was with, the Important People in My Life, people who were invariably women or gay men. If someone interesting or attractive came my way, I ignored him. And I practiced Having a Life. My life was rich, full, I told myself frequently. After all, I had friends, a career, interests, hobbies, a vibrator.

This same friend later admonished me, while we sat at a sports bar near Wrigley Field, that it was no wonder I wasn't meeting anyone, since I ignored all the men around me. "That guy wanted to buy you a drink and you didn't even bother to thank him," she said, pointing to a man whose T-shirt rode as high as his jeans rode low.

The bar was one that my friend, now happily married to Jim, would never have ventured into except that she had decided I needed help in finding a husband. Called Sluggers, it attracts a clientele whose idea of a good read is a Miller label. Even so, I was racked with guilt. It's true, I thought. I *don't* give anyone a chance. I'm too judgmental, I cling to stereotypes, and, I admitted, I keep a mental checklist.

I tried to keep my checklist to the basics—good sense of humor, likes travel, books, and the outdoors. But still, I knew, I really wanted a Bill Murray/Rhett Butler/Ivy League professor composite who also was down-to-earth and an expert skier. At least I had no salary requirements or nose-size stipulations like other women I knew. Still, maybe I was being too choosy. I tossed out my list. And so began my Open to Dating period. I vowed to give everyone a chance, no matter what he looked like or what his interests, priorities, and values were. I said yes to everyone.

This was different from my open period in college. Back then, I thought that the more parties I went to, and the more time I spent in bars, the greater the chances of meeting my destiny. More realistically, alcohol gave me confidence and made me daring and witty—or so I believed. It also made me slur my words and gave me a beer belly. I did not date a whole lot during this period.

Now, however, I dated constantly. I listened attentively, caringly, to long tales of betrayal by former wives. I went to hardware shows and Bob Seger concerts. I attended lectures by obscure, rhyming poets. I let someone I barely knew dress me up as a stick-woman for a Halloween costume contest he was sadly convinced we would win. I always smiled and said I had a nice time at the end of my dates. Inevitably, however, I failed to make a graceful exit, jumping out of the car too quickly or saying good-bye through a tight crack in the door.

I grew tired of my dismal pretense, and I grew tired of the time I was spending away from my life. There had to be another way.

I started sneaking into the Getting a Husband section of the bookstore to check out new arrivals. Treat it like a job search, one book said, taking a practical approach. You take your career seriously, why not love? Make a résumé for your soul-mate search, the author instructed. State your objective clearly, list your past experience and pertinent education. Treat dates like job interviews. Investigate his background, talk to his friends, read books on his interests. Ask him, "What do you have to offer me that other men do not? Do you offer extra benefits, such as the use of your Porsche or skill as a masseur?"

I read *Cosmo*. Those women might be insipid, I reasoned, but they always have men. Get *out* there, the magazine exhorted. Join clubs, volunteer, exercise regularly, pay compliments often, memorize jokes, and wear plenty of *feral* clothing! I looked at the fashion and beauty pages, and bought lipstick, nail polish, perfume, eyeliner, eye shadow, eyelid cream, an eyelash curler, and an eyelash separator. I bought more revealing clothing. I bought sexy lingerie so that I would always feel sultry. I bought hats.

I watched segments of *Oprah* on topics such as "Women who think too much about worrying about not having a man." The men on Oprah said every woman they knew just wanted to get married. They felt like trophies. They said if they ever met a woman who didn't want to get married they would marry her right away. This sounded like most of the men I know. They are irrevocably convinced that all most women want to do is get married to whoever will take them, and if they open the door a crack—by, say, taking you to *Terminator 2*—you will burst through it in an armor-plated wedding dress, run them over with a station wagon, and immobilize them in fresh sod.

I told men who asked that I wasn't certain whether I wanted to get married. I told this to so many men and relatives and friends that I began to believe it myself, even though I suspected I would change my mind if I met the right man. The usual expert with a degree told the women on *Oprah* that their real problem was that they really didn't want to get married, so they avoided long-term relationships. I decided that was my problem. I am afraid of commitment, I thought, so I intentionally seek out commitment-shy men and force them to commit so I won't have to.

I began to wonder if I was too possessive, even though I possessed no one. I wondered if I didn't express my needs clearly enough, even though there was no one clamoring to hear them. One day I decided I was passive-aggressive, and the next that I was aggressive-passive. I concluded that I was passive-passive on some days and aggressive-aggressive on others.

I was not unhappy, but I was growing increasingly lonely and I was tired of my lust and of satisfying it on unsatisfying men. I listened with amazement when women told me that sometimes they got tired of having sex with their boyfriends or husbands. There were many nights when they just wanted to read, they said. I longed to be so saturated and satiated that I actually might say no. I might say, "Tomorrow, honey. *The Simpsons* are on."

I was tired of having sex. I wanted to make love.

And let's face it—life is far richer with passion and romance or at least someone to come home and watch the news with. The arrogance of men who think all women want to marry them infuriates me as much as the naivete of women who believe a wedding day will solve their problems. But I began to admit that I did want to get married, even that I probably wanted to have children, although the ticking of my biological clock was barely audible.

I wish I could say I solved my troubles by ignoring the

media and the advice of my friends. I wish I could say that I truly decided I was a wonderful woman, that I gained the confidence to believe in myself, and that men consequently flocked to my side. Instead, I met a wonderful man. I am convinced I deserve him because I was patient. "You just have to be patient," I tell all my single friends. "There are plenty of good men out there."

I just wish I knew whether I found him because I stopped looking or I stopped looking because I found him.

Conquest

MAGDA KRANCE

It happens unexpectedly. I see someone and I simply must have him. Not forever, but just for long enough to know that I've gotten him. Not necessarily in bed, although sometimes that would be nice. Not because I don't love my husband, and not because he doesn't satisfy me—I do, he does. Just for the sport of it, the pure pleasure of conquest. I have followed men, casually calculated and maneuvered to cross paths, to bump at the elevator or the ski-lift line or while boarding the bus. Sometimes, an exchanged look is enough, or a few mumbled pleasantries. Sometimes it's not.

An established relationship, marriage or otherwise, is the staple of emotional life. A conquest is the occasional dollop of caviar, the rare truffle, the exquisite champagne. It doesn't last. It wasn't meant to. Ah, but it's delicious, special, forbidden, dangerous but not deadly, not usually, if you're careful.

Men do this, of course, always have. Not all of them, of course, but plenty. And so do women, some of us, anyway. Nice girls aren't supposed to chase; they're supposed to wait, to demur, to be the objects of desire. But pursuit is fun, as men and dogs and cats and other predatory creatures have known for ages. It's sport. It recharges the batteries and strokes the ego. And when desire sparks, we're entitled to enjoy the pursuit, too.

Not that most women are as ham-handed about it as men can be. We scuff over our tracks, let the unwitting objects of our desire think that they noticed us first—usually, but not always. Sometimes it's fun to let them in on the secret, to tell them they've been stalked. Some are flattered, pleased at the reversal of stereotypical roles. Others are alarmed, even confused, as if their manliness were threatened, as if they'd complimented your fragrance and you'd told them it was men's cologne.

A man who's a friend of mine, a veteran pursuer, tells me I'm more male than female, because I'm more like him than like the women he targets. It would threaten his hypermasculine self-image to acknowledge that women can enjoy the thrill of the chase as much as men. When we talk it's guy to guy. When he remembers that we're not on the same side of the sex fence, he's rattled.

Although I'm thinking in the present tense here, the moments that inspired these thoughts are all securely embedded in the past. To say things have changed profoundly is an understatement. It used to be that, when conquest crossed our minds, male or female, we didn't have to be all that careful. We practically didn't have to think at all, once birth control became easily available. We could just do it, fly off the edge of attraction and not worry about landing. It was a lot like recreational drugs, which mostly look pretty stupid and dangerous now from the perspective of maturity, but which seemed like a lot of fun at the time. We did a lot of stupid things in the name of lust, but we had a lot of fun discovering ourselves and others in the process.

In the end, though, it's the process that's usually the best part. I'm experienced enough to know that a lot of times the wanting is better than the having. The pursuit is almost always more exhilarating than the conquest.

Crying

LAURIE ABRAHAM

When I received word that my grandmother had died hundreds of miles away in a cool hospital room in late July, Mike let me lie on top of him and cry. With the bed shuddering in concert with the semis that nightly rumbled into the city outside my window, I wept. I mourned that I had not seen my grandmother since Christmas, that she would not see me marry, that I would never again linger as I held her, feeling our bodies tall against each other, proud that I alone in my family shared her five feet, seven inches of height.

After my tears slowed, I became aware of Mike's body under mine, and I stretched to match my knees to his knees, to curl my feet around his ankles, to press my chest to his. I slept.

That night is memorable not only because I lost someone who was dear but because it was one of the few times in a

year and a half with Mike when he has comforted me through
a long cry. Writing about crying is fraught with perils. An
essay I wrote about my sadness after a breakup prompted a
writing instructor to warn me to "discern the boundary between grief and indulgent self-pity." For good prose's sake, I
agree that such a line must be drawn, so I tread uneasily into
this risky territory. But tread I must, because I fear that if
my eyes are ever dry for Mike my heart may follow.

In a world where crying is equated with weakness or deception (the latter charge, of course, is usually leveled at
women), it's not easy to weep with abandon. But when I rise
to the occasion, when I let tears run their natural course instead of swallowing them in an effort to regain "adult" compo-
sure, I feel exquisitely refreshed. Crying serves the same
unburdening purpose as confession, absolving my mistakes
and washing away some of life's inevitable disappointments
and failures. It emboldens me to move on.

Mike, of course, has never ordered me not to cry. We've
discussed this topic several times and he's told me to feel free
to cry. But the way he has responded when I've barely whim-
pered makes me wary. Sometimes in bed, after we've made
love, I can feel my eyes gloss with tears. It's often after I've
had a rotten week, when hurts big and small have piled up,
and I feel like letting go. I don't think he always notices the
intimation of tears, but at other times, I'm sure he does. He
too deliberately rolls away from me in bed; my tears seem to
make him nervous. Several mornings when I've been on the
verge of tears after our lovemaking, I've sensed Mike counting
the minutes until he could escape. He's too polite to leap out
of bed immediately after we finish, but after several minutes
he jumps up. "Let's get dressed," he says, pulling his jeans
on as fast as a fireman responding to an alarm. I feel embarrassed saying, "Stay, I need to cry." So before I know it,
Mike is humming in the kitchen making coffee, and I'm sulk-
ing beneath the sheets.

Writing this makes my throat clot with tears and at the same time makes me want to laugh. Many times over, I've heard couples observe that the things they most loved about each other are the things they end up resenting. As it is with me and Mike. His relentless cheerfulness is one of the things I most admire about him; he can be a joy. But at the same time, I regret the lack of empathy that sometimes accompanies his unflagging optimism.

During one of our more honest exchanges, Mike asked me how I could expect him to respect my tears when he's not comfortable with his own. Good question. I know that Mike expends significant energy trying to maintain good karma, and my sadness threatens to upset the fragile truce he has struck with his emotions. I told him recently that after watching a television show about a woman dying of cancer, I felt lucky that my problems were so small. Mike readily identified. For me, this grateful feeling only lasted a half hour; reviewing the world's horrors in my head accompanied by the refrain "just look at how lucky I am" has never truly relieved my sorrow. But Mike told me that those kinds of comparisons undergird his positive outlook on life.

We are very different. The difference matters because it saps our intimacy. Holding my tears in check makes me feel distant from Mike, as though I cannot share myself with him. Mike evidently feels as close to me as he needs to during sex, but that's not enough for me.

I have tried to talk myself out of this need for Mike's shoulder to cry on. What do you want? I ask myself. Not only does Mike make my heart beat faster, but he's intelligent, ambitious, romantic. Cry by yourself, I tell myself. So I lie on my bed, a few sobs issue forth, and the next thing I know I'm reading a book, forcing my thoughts to travel elsewhere. Or I go into the bathroom and sit on the toilet, but soon I'm up, staring at my ugly, red eyes in the mirror. (I challenge anyone to continue crying while watching herself in a mirror.)

Though crying alone is a surefire way to dry up my tears, my sadness only festers. What I want is the real release that comes when I have a witness to my tears, someone to slowly rub my back and say, "There, there." When I don't cry at home, tears threaten to erupt in the most inappropriate places. Though I've never broken down at work—and never plan to— I've been close enough that I've adjourned to the washroom to pull myself together. If I cleared the decks more often in private, perhaps a thoughtless remark by my boss would not trigger an unconscious cataloging of every such slight that had gone before.

I've considered relieving Mike of this responsibility and going to my friends for comfort, but I do not have the kind of relationships with women that allow easy tears. Though I may sound like a sobbing fool, I have cast myself as the strong and capable one in many of my friendships. That may change one day; I'd like at least one female friend whom I'd trust to rock me through a long cry. But that's really beside the point. I want Mike's solace, his understanding, more than anyone else's.

I also wonder whether it would be enough if Mike felt comfortable comforting me. Do I also need him to reciprocate and soak my shirt? Once, undone by the stress of finishing his post-doctoral work, Mike cried for a few minutes and let me hold him. I felt close to him and hoped I was helping, but he has not offered a repeat performance. Sometimes I feel as if that's all his crying would be, a performance, in response to my nagging him to share more of his emotions with me. He told me once that he sobs every time he hears Bruce Springsteen's "The River." What I thought but did not say was that I hope I'm with him sometime when the song comes on the radio; I want to know whether his version of "sobbing" turns out to be tears in the corners of his eyes. Sadness is such uncharted terrain between us.

On the other hand, although we women for years have

been begging our men to express their emotions, if mine prefers not to be vulnerable around me, perhaps I shouldn't
whine about it. Mike says tears don't help him much, and the
purpose of his crying shouldn't be to make me feel better. I
cannot command him to cry. Sometimes I wonder whether
men are less capable than women of finding a middle ground
between stoicism and emotional cataclysm. Their fear that one
tear will unleash an unceasing flood is apparently so much
stronger than ours. One male friend insists that women delude
themselves when they imagine that they want their men to
cry. We've all grown up in the same culture, he says, and
both sexes perceive men's tears as a weakness that they would
just as soon not know about.

What is the price of my unspent tears? Pondering this
question makes me think back to the woman on TV dying of
cancer. My tears obviously will not cure her, nor will they
forge world peace, or build homes for the homeless. Their use
is small and self-serving. A good cry clears the way for a good
laugh, for good sex, even. Tears are one way to nourish an
oasis of love in a sometimes barren land.

My Son

LAURA GREEN

The summer my son Nicholas turned fourteen, he began thinking about girls and relationships in a way that told me "I can't avoid this anymore." That was the summer girls started calling the house in the evening, girls I had never seen, girls from faraway neighborhoods I'd never heard of. Their voices were pleasant and admirably straightforward. They never wanted to leave their names, but it didn't matter. Nick always knew who was calling.

My son is a good-looking boy, confident and quirky. So far, girls have liked him and, so far, he has brushed them aside a bit dismissively. So how he thinks about girls and how he will treat them has been on my mind. I want him to be honest, considerate, straightforward, articulate, reasonable in his expectations, ready to go halfway—all the things I think are necessary in a mate. Since his sense of what it is to be a man is far from formed, I think I have a chance to get the message across. So far I haven't been too successful, which may explain why I got so mad at both Nick and my husband in a restaurant one night.

It was a summer night on Long Island, and the neighborhood restaurant was crowded. At most of the tables, the talk buzzed of boats. Our town lies between two deep harbors on Long Island Sound and boats are as much a part of its life as third cars for the kids. A young man in a booth across from our table leaned over and kissed his girlfriend. Then, as Nick watched, he offered her his hand to help her through the ordeal of getting out of the booth, steered her to the door with an authoritative, possessive hand on her shoulder, and tucked her into his car. Like something out of the fifties.

The cars here are from the fifties, too. Chryslers big as ocean liners, Cadillacs, long station wagons. If it weren't for the in-your-face Mercedeses and aggressive little Jaguars outside the dry cleaners and carry-out stores, you could believe that people still coveted American cars. Some of the women's cars have license-plate frames that say things like "Spoiled rotten and loving every minute of it." It is a part of the country where women seem to expect men to hold open doors, push them out to the car, and make lots of money. After twenty years in Chicago, it is a strange place to be.

The girls look different here than they do back home, like something from the fifties, only with more money. Do you remember Bob and Justine from *American Bandstand*? Like Justine, the girls have big finger-in-the-socket hair. It stands several inches high in front, moussed up around combs, clamps, and other armatures. Their nails are long and manicured. They prefer jeans with ruffles and bows. They wear noticeable earrings, mostly dangly and filigreed. They carry themselves like great prizes.

These girls have been noticing Nick. Women have, too. At the Cub Scout picnic, of all places, a pretty blond in her twenties asked him to play tennis with her after watching him on the court. The two of them played a hard game while his best friend watched on the sidelines.

That night in the restaurant, Nick asked us a good question. "What is thought?" It quickly came around to matters of perception and that's when my husband brought up The Study.

For the last twenty years, my husband has periodically

talked about The Study, to my increasing irritation. This study is as evasive as fog. I've never read it, never read about it, never heard anyone else discuss it. Though it may exist nowhere but his mind, to my husband the study is very real. A classic in its field, he assures me. What it boils down to is this. Psychologists build a room with funny angles and a tilted floor. The warped room affects the viewer's sense of proportion so that people walking across it seem to get smaller as they come closer. (Never mind that the very idea of this room strains credibility. For the story's sake, let's just assume these psychologists also were experts in funhouse construction.)

As I fidgeted with my bread, my husband told Nick about the room. "Every observer said the people got littler when they should have been bigger," he said, his voice animated. "Then, guess what happened next?"

"What?" said Nick, fascinated, his spaghetti and meatballs growing cold.

My husband leaned across the table. "Then they had a new bride watch her husband cross the room. Rather than let him appear small, she said that the room grew bigger! You know why?"

Nick shook his head. He looked as rapt as the students in the photos in college catalogs.

"Because he was so important to her that she could not let him be small. She distorted the room instead!"

He smiled. Nick smiled, too, the two of them smug and happy in their apparent superiority over the poor, manipulated bride. I smiled, too. And then I said, "If I hear that story one more time, I am going to throw up!"

Bewilderment. Surprise. Annoyance.

"What's that all about?" my husband asked. Every couple has signal words, words that mean trouble is coming. When Steve says, "What's that all about?" he means, "What is this convoluted feminist bullshit you are forcing on me?"

So we got into it. "I am sick of that story. All it says

is that men think they have to be the center of a woman's universe."

"I didn't say that at all. I was talking about perception."

"Whose? Yours or the psychologists'? Do you bend reality to make me look bigger?"

"What's that got to do with it?"

"Yeah, Mom, you don't understand," added Nick, rushing to defend his father. "It's about the way people see things."

"It's about the way men see women, Nick. It's about their fantasies about women."

He looked at Steve. Steve looked at him. I am the odd one out in their eyes, the voice of female irrationality, of emotionalism, of hostility to, pardon the expression, science. Almost always in the past, Nick was my ally in arguments, whether or not I wanted his earnest assistance. Time and again he took my side in fights with his older sister and father, who are both hard as flint when they are angry. He defended me with the bravery of wholehearted love.

That night in the restaurant, he was no longer my little boy but his father's son and one of the guys. That is part of growing up, I know, and it's hard for me to let go, not just because he is my youngest, but because I can see my influence ebbing away. The more my husband and I argued, the more upset and defensive my son became. This wasn't helping him figure out what to expect from a woman. It wasn't helping at all. I was critical of men's expectations and that suddenly meant I was critical of his wishes, even if they weren't fully formed. That his opinion might be what we were fighting over didn't occur to me until much later.

Ostensibly sticking to the study, I asked, "If it's such a good study did they have any new grooms watch their wives walk across the room? Did the wives get bigger or smaller?"

"What's that all about?"

"Everything. Why do you always talk about that one woman?"

"Because she proves a story about perception . . ."

"Men's perceptions. If it's about anything at all, it's about men's perceptions of a perfect wife."

"No it isn't. But he's so important to her that she had to do that to keep her world rational."

"Oh, for God's sake!"

We went on for about fifteen minutes, stopping only because Nick was getting upset. My husband promised to find The Study. He won't. I'm convinced it doesn't exist. It's scientific nonsense and about as valid as planting beans by the light of the moon.

More to the point, I don't want my son to buy into this foolishness. If he wants that kind of devotion, he should get a spaniel. It is enough for someone to want to be with you and to prefer your company more often than not. Wives prove their love by keeping a straight face when their husbands think they are dying of summer colds, by sexual loyalty, by gladly embracing their in-laws, by being friends. That's plenty. Only a psychologist who builds funhouses would ask a woman to sacrifice the reality of her perceptions.

As Steve and I picked sullenly at our desserts, Nick watched our waitress. She was probably a college student, thin, fresh, enthusiastic, and efficient. Her long red hair was the real thing, not a mousse job. It quivered about her head in an amazing, curly aurora. If she watched a man walk across a stage, I thought, she would never distort him. She would see him as he is.

She looked sensible and for a moment I wanted to ask her opinion of The Study. But I didn't. What if she didn't get it? And besides, I'm not ready for Nick to listen to her, or to Steve, for that matter. When it comes to women, I want him to listen, with that great loyalty he once felt, to me.

Peace

MAGDA KRANCE

We don't fight.

I don't want to sound smug or self-righteous, but it's true.

It can sometimes be embarrassing to admit—not because I would want to fight with my husband, but because fighting seems to be a fact of life, a given, for so many couples, including a few we know. They don't seem to question the fact that they fight; some even boast about it. It's part of the fabric of their relationships, even something they'd miss if it wasn't there. Perhaps it helps define them. Some almost seem proud describing a particularly surly row, with a sort of "Boy, I sure showed him/her!" swagger.

When people I know talk about fighting, I feel curious and bewildered. Do they yell loud enough to wake the children? the neighbors? What is it they say in the heat of the moment? Do they ever slap or slug each other? Throw things? Threaten divorce? Make wild love afterwards? Or sleep in separate rooms? Buy expensive gifts to make up? I'm not sure whether I want to know those kinds of details about people I like. I don't ask.

And if I mention that we don't fight, the conversation often goes cold with disbelief, as if there's something wrong with my husband and me, as if we don't belong to the club, as if our emotions must be horribly suppressed and ready to burst.

They're not; we're not. For the most part, our life together is harmonious. We get along very well, plain and simple. We do so by negotiating and conceding. Over the years we've gotten into the habit of taking turns acquiescing to each other's piques. One asserts, the other acquiesces. Each makes requests. Each takes orders. Neither has absolute authority.

Oh sure, we sometimes toss off little insults facetiously when we're peeved—sort of shooting blanks verbally. At times we bicker and whine, we quibble and bitch, we snap and sulk. We blow off our steam a little at a time, instead of exploding in each other's face. Our disagreements are few and generally petty, mostly pertaining to little domestic matters—a dirty spoon left on the kitchen counter, lax table manners, whether the baby should be quick-rinsed in the sink or bathed in the tub—things like that. The disagreements seldom escalate.

We tend to get annoyed more than angry, and annoyance isn't that hard to work through and get past in a hurry. It's a cloudburst, and then it clears. It's usually about small stuff, and we're usually archly polite about the offense, albeit with a cutting edge: *Please* don't leave your shoes in the living room. *Please* clean the cutting board when you're done with it. Would you *please* close the door when you're using the bathroom. *Next* time, *please* turn off the television if you're not going to be in the room. *Thank* you.

I'll admit that sometimes I spoil for a reason to get mad at Steve. Sometimes I need to be provoked into a good cry because of PMS, or because of stresses and frustrations from the world outside our marriage. I'll find myself needling him about one thing or another until he snaps or barks at me (usually justifiably), at which point I'll start crying, at which point he'll feel bad for making me feel bad (even though I made him do it), and we'll hug and snuffle and apologize to each other for our thoughtless or irrational behavior. That's about as bad as it gets. And, I'm happy to realize, it's happening a lot less than it used to.

I never learned how to fight. It was something my parents simply didn't do. They expressed love, affection, and hospitality freely and generously, and the rest was genteel coexistence. If they had grown-up matters to discuss, they did it in Polish, their native language—but their voices never became even remotely shrill or threatening. What went on between them never alarmed me, never made me worry or feel insecure. Most of what little I knew about fighting I learned from flamboyant movie and television images of marital combat. The rest I picked up in the homes of some childhood playmates whose parents sparred in what seemed like vitriolic terms, and from my oldest brother and his then wife.

My brother is basically a nice, quiet guy, but his twenty-five-year marriage brought out the worst in both him and his wife. In their mostly miserable years together they both drank, smoked, and brooded heavily. She relentlessly needled him till he rose to the bait. The air in their home was always thick with tension, resentment, anger, bitterness, and unhappiness. They fought over their daughter, and used her against each other. Visiting them was hellish; they truly evoked the viciousness of Liz Taylor and Richard Burton in *Who's Afraid of Virginia Woolf?* We would get together for ostensibly happy occasions—birthdays, Thanksgiving, Christmas—that would inevitably disintegrate into combative misery for them and acute discomfort for the rest of us. And yet they clung together, the fear of life alone more desperate than their hate.

Finally, though, my brother left. He called us on a Friday night, asking to come stay with us awhile. He fairly percolated with pent-up resentment and relief and anxiety about what to do next—where to live, how to balance his checkbook, how to manage. Six weeks later, amazingly, he met the love of his life. They married two years after that. But that's another story.

My first couple of years in college, a guy named Ken was my best friend. We would be getting along fine for a few weeks, and then he'd turn peevish and critical. He was spoiling for a fight—something he just needed to do—but I had no clue what was happening. I would earnestly agree with his severe assessments of my flaws and promise to improve myself, and then he'd yell at me for being such a patsy, and what was wrong with me, anyway? Why didn't I defend myself against his criticism? Why didn't I fight back?

To me, the whole exchange was dumbfounding. Fighting for the sake of fighting? What was the point?

There can be something liberating about it, I suppose, even exhilarating, but the prospect of entering a serious fight— with anyone—terrifies me. Sure, I imagine things I'd *like* to say to someone who aggravates me, but I can't bear the thought of the consequences of confrontation—what would the object of my anger say back? And wouldn't that be worse?

So maybe I am repressed. Fighting seems to be a matter of spontaneous combustion, and I go to pieces anticipating fights that won't happen because I won't put myself in a position to let them happen. I like to think of my avoidance behavior as the emotional equivalent of defensive driving.

But is that so bad? Isn't peaceful coexistence instead of combativeness what leading a civilized life is supposed to be about?

Consider the horrifying statistics on domestic violence— abuse and murder in the name of what was supposed to be love. Would the incidence of such violence be as high if our society hadn't fallen into the horrible habit of accepting and even condoning violence (especially through television and film) as a means of resolving personal conflict? Where verbal violence is tolerated and accepted, physical violence follows far too easily and too often.

That's nothing I want in my life. Which is why, I guess, we don't fight.

Sleeping Alone

JANICE ROSENBERG

From across the cabin the single bed beckoned. Beside me in the standard double my husband Michael wheezed and snored, victim of a summer cold caught on the first day of our vacation in Grand Teton National Park. Not the neatest sleeper in the best of health or the largest bed, my husband had managed to mummify himself in the covers, leaving me with only six inches of thin sheet and scratchy blanket. You can hardly divorce a man for this, but if a cold was ruining his vacation, sleepless nights were about to ruin mine.

Stealthily I left his side. Why did I feel as if I were heading out for Brazil? I swept clothes and coins and hiking-trail brochures from the single bed and turned the covers back in a deep smooth fold. I took off my nightgown and got in naked. The sheets were cool and tightly tucked. Lying on my stomach, I worked my feet along the edges of the mattress, loosening the covers. Then I hooked one foot over each side and stretched my arms, marking the territory as mine, all mine. In the chilly room with the covers nearly over my head I thought of bunk beds in camp cabins. Branches brushed against the window above my head. Crickets sounded in the surrounding forest. I shivered rapturously and shut my eyes.

What was it about these pleasures that seemed so forbidden? I'll come right to the point. After twenty-two years of

happy if not quite blissful marriage I'm feeling a dangerous
yearning: I think—no, I'm positive—that I like sleeping alone.

I don't know how many movies I've seen where couples
sleep the night away entwined in each other's limbs and a
tangle of unhealthy-looking sheets. In *Sea of Love* Ellen Barkin
and Al Pacino don't even know each other and already they're
willing to share a sweaty space. It's sexy on the screen but I
can never believe it happens in real life.

The last time Michael and I slept that close was in a twin
bed before we were married. Neither of us got much sleep and
sometime near dawn we each realized the other was awake.
To pass the time Michael sang Donovan's then-popular song
"Mellow Yellow." I had never heard the phrase "elec-trical
banana" and lying there in his musty dorm room I thought it
was a riot.

When we married, like all our friends, we bought a queen-
sized bed. My parents and his had slept in the fifties' answer
to the standard double—twin beds pushed together under a
shared headboard. Although we couldn't imagine our parents
"doing it" (much less liking it), we agreed that their twin beds
would certainly have cut down on spontaneity if and when
they did.

But all the same, from the beginning, I created my own
sleeping space. Over the years it's been rare for us to touch
in the middle of the night, let alone embrace, let even more
alone make love. And I know the choice was mine. In the
middle of the night, if I sensed that he was awake, I kept my
back turned and breathed in a sleeping rhythm. If he reached
for my hand, I curled my fingers lifelessly in his, then slipped
away. Michael gradually accepted this, trained unconsciously
the way I trained him not to hang his coat on my side of the
front-hall closet. (Writing this, I feel the lack of generosity in
both these instances and wish I were different.)

Because lovemaking in the middle of the night is so rare
for us, when it does happen (when I let myself let it happen)

there's a dreamy sensuality about it that is special. If only I
could remember in between how much I like it. Most recently,
suffering from jet lag on a visit to Israel, suddenly wide awake
at 2 a.m., we made love. Afterwards, warmed and relaxed,
we fell instantly back to sleep.

As for sleeping alone, I envy married women who travel
on business. A few months after our Grand Teton vacation
(where, by the way, I slept in that single bed every night),
for the first time ever, I had work to do out of town. The
town was small and boring, but that was okay. As I packed
my bag I actually looked forward to the independence of a
night by myself in a hotel. In a Holiday Inn in a small town!
When the evening meeting I had come to cover ended, I
bought a beer at a drive-through liquor store and a bag of
chips at a 7-Eleven, and, feeling resourceful, took them to my
room. I tuned the TV to a late-night talk show and got into
bed. At home I never want to watch late-night talk shows.
The commercials make me crazy. Alone in a hotel it was the
right thing to do.

That night, for the first time ever, I slept on Michael's
side of the bed. Sleeping in my usual prone position, I liked
knowing there was an entire field of linen to my right. Without him there sighing, snoring, turning, getting up to blow
his nose, the covers remained neatly drawn up over me. The
silent pitch-black room invited dreams, sexy ones.

It had happened before. A couple of years ago on the
morning after a highly stimulating writers' conference, I woke
at 5 a.m. Thoughts swirled madly through my sleepy brain.
Desperate to be alone with those thoughts, I dragged a pillow
and blanket down to the basement couch. In the coal-mine-
dark room I dozed and dreamed. It seemed to me that, upstairs, Michael's presence had interfered with those dreams,
as if his body blocked signals from the other side. I woke
inspired to write a dozen stories.

When I came home from my business trip, I asked Michael

if he had missed me. He paused just long enough to make me think he too had found some pleasure in sleeping alone. With a self-satisfied grin he told me he watched a movie right up to the very end, tuned in David Letterman, then fell asleep in the center of the bed with the TV still on. And, he added, to tease me, in the morning the covers were in an ungodly disarray.

So, when our older son went away to college, did I take over his single-bedded room where no television commercials would keep me awake? Or barring such total isolation, did I campaign for those old twin beds pushed together? Did I even go as far as to suggest we trade in our queen-size for a king and the illusion of separate sleep?

Naaa. I didn't do any of those things. Sure, one part of me wants to be alone, but a much bigger part of me wants to sleep next to Michael. It's warm and snuggly and luxurious and reassuring to know that he's there. I need that knowledge more than the precisely folded cool morning sheets of a single bed. Perhaps I always will.

The Red Velvet Dress

LAURIE ABRAHAM

I played catch with my father from the time I was eight; he hung a basketball net over our driveway when I was ten, and when I was fourteen he told me, only half joking, that one way to keep other girls from rebounding was to step on their feet. He also told me I could go anywhere for college (anywhere in the Midwest, it turned out) and that all professions were open to me. Thanks to my father, I learned to trust my mind and my jump shot. Yet I wanted him to do one more thing for me. I yearn for a memory that doesn't exist: I am twirling about in a red velvet dress, long blond curls flying, and suddenly my father scoops me up. "You are the prettiest little girl in the world," he says, his face close to mine.

When I read of a woman whose father called her "princess," or told her she was the most beautiful little girl in the world, I feel cheated, jealous, wistful for what I have missed. I imagine this woman's face and body to be the opposite of mine: She has straight black hair, dark eyes, full lips, and round breasts. Even if she does not meet that physical ideal, I know she must feel gorgeous; her father willed it. She is the woman who is held up as an example in women's magazines: "Jackie isn't beautiful by traditional standards, but she never spends Saturday nights eating yogurt in front of the TV. She believes she's sexy, and men respond to that." I am certain Jackie's father told her she was beautiful.

I am embarrassed by the importance I ascribe to these
words. In public, I have only disdain for the way our worth,
women's worth, continues to be measured by how we look.
But in private, I still want to be one of the chosen ones—
chosen by men, that is. As a child, I was never "Daddy's
little girl." Instead, I *was* Daddy: aggressive, athletic, volatile.
"Thankfully," my mother informed me in grade school, "you
did not end up looking like him." It wasn't really him that
she worried about—my father is a good-looking man—but his
female incarnation, his older sister. I was born with her square
jaw and fair skin tending toward ruddiness, but somehow the
sum of the parts was not the same. Photographs tell me that
today I indeed favor my mother, but I have never stopped
feeling secretly pleased when someone notices that we look
alike. I remember how grateful I felt as a thirteen-year-old
when a woman at church told my mother and me that we
shared the same "peachy complexions." My only sister usually
collected the peaches-and-cream compliments. Even now I feel
proud when strangers say to my mother and me, "You two
must be related."

For years I doubted my appeal to men, specifically my sex
appeal. Studies of young girls have shown they are as confident and bold as boys until they reach early adolescence,
about age twelve. Then they start noticing how older girls
criticize their own bodies, too flat or fat, how they defer to
boys and try to curry male approval. It is in this milieu that
every girl grows up, but some enter the fray with a stronger
sense of self-worth than others, and so eventually return to
trusting themselves. For me, however, the gawky thirteen-
year-old with long legs, no curves, braces, and wire-framed
glasses never quite grew up and left home. She is the part of
me who dated the same boy-man from her senior prom to her
twenty-fifth birthday, at least partly because she thought no
one else would want her. I ended the relationship only after

another man pursued me relentlessly; even I couldn't deny that he was interested.

Though I know these days that I am far from ugly, that I could even be considered attractive, I tend to qualify my looks: not bad for an intelligent woman, not bad if you like women who are pretty in an unusual way, or who don't stand out in a crowd. Such qualifiers explain why the comments my father *did* make about my looks, while well-intentioned, did not give me what I needed. The shortcomings of "That's an attractive dress" or "You look nice tonight" are obvious: Take off the dress, change the night, and what's left?

After the breakup with my longtime boyfriend, and before I got involved in another serious relationship, I had a small epiphany: Men, all kinds of them, wanted to date me. I juggled four at once and felt like a queen. One date, for instance, told me that he'd liked me even before he noticed the way I moved. He noticed the way Laurie Kaye Abraham moved? I thought she merely walked. Incredible! Wonderful! Thank you, Roger! Another man asked me out while standing next to the cauliflower at the grocery store. That I had nothing in common with him was irrelevant. My friends couldn't believe that in this dangerous world I'd go out with someone I met over vegetables, but caution had no place during this experimental phase.

Though that experience made me more sure of myself, I am still troubled by a lack of confidence about my appeal, especially when it comes to the arena where looks matter most: sex. I too often do not have the fortitude to ask for what I want, or refuse what I don't.

That fact became all too clear at the beginning of my last relationship. I did not want to have sex with Todd when he pulled me into the woods on our third date, but I was sure he would lose interest if I declined. A few dates later I had begun to enjoy sleeping with him, with one important qualification: I feared I might get pregnant. But I did not have the guts to interrupt and put in the diaphragm that I had just visited the doctor to get, and I could not ask Todd to use a condom. My reticence about asking for condoms is especially indefensible, as I wrote news stories on AIDS for several years and have hosted two house parties to encourage women like me to practice safe sex.

Obviously, a fear of rejection so strong that it would reconcile me to risking unplanned pregnancy or worse is more complicated than my father's not noticing me in a red velvet dress. What I missed from my father, or from my mother for that matter, was gloriously prejudiced, unqualified, that-girl-can-do-no-wrong approval, the kind that fills your cup to running over, the kind that pushes you out to meet the world believing you deserve to be loved. Had I heard my father say I was beautiful, I might have been able to exert a bit of extra courage and grace with men I would later meet. At the very least, it would have been thrilling to hear those words. I'm sure of that because lately my stepfather has been saying what my father never could, and I'm reveling in it.

One evening recently my mother called me from a pay phone in a crowded restaurant; I was struggling to stay away from a dangerous relationship, and she wanted to support me. The phone was near their table. At the end of the conversation, she said, "Your stepfather told me to tell you you're beautiful."

"Why?" I asked. "What's he talking about?"

"That's all he said," she replied. I hung up the phone smiling, and I didn't call the man I knew I shouldn't.

A few weeks later I called home, again worked up about the man I was trying to avoid. My mom was not there, so my stepfather and I began talking. After a while, he told me that he understood why this man kept calling me, even though I had insisted I would not see him until he broke up with his longtime girlfriend. Most men would feel lucky to date a woman like you, he said. You are intelligent, well-read. He cleared his throat. "And I would imagine that men must find

you very attractive." He said this plainly but then sounded
flustered. He seemed to be thinking that telling one's step-
daughter she is very attractive is precariously close to inappro-
priateness, and, I'm sure he thought, liable to dangerous
misinterpretation. "Of course I can't really say that, being
your stepfather," he mumbled quickly. From my perspective,
though, his being my stepfather made him just the man for
the job.

COMPLICATIONS

Love and Need

Years ago I read *The Art of Loving* by psychoanalyst Erich Fromm. He said you should need someone because you love him, not love him because you need him. The former is mature love, he said, the latter, dependency.

For a long time I tried very hard to convince myself I believed this neat appraisal and to act on it, to love my husband, Michael, in some pure realm beyond the fray of everyday life. I wasn't very successful and I think it's because the matter isn't as clear cut as that.

The close connection between need and love became apparent to me during the tense period when our friends Fran and Sid were getting divorced. Fran and I were having lunch when she leaned toward me across the table, clearly struck by the wonder of her own epiphany. *When they married, she had "only thought" she loved Sid.* In other words, she hadn't really loved him at all. No wonder she didn't love him "anymore"! That reminded me of a conversation I'd once overheard between my mother and a woman whose daughter had recently broken her engagement. "She only thought she loved him," the woman said.

At the time, I meditated on this simple sentence as if it were the complete works of Plato. How does *thinking* you love someone differ from actually loving someone? I suppose the mother meant she herself hadn't thought the engagement would last. But had the daughter also had doubts? I wished I could ask her. If she'd had doubts, then okay, maybe she did "only think" she was in love. But if she'd had no doubts— heard bells, walked on air, spent hours gazing into his eyes— didn't that mean she *did* love him?

When I was in ninth grade my friends and I talked a lot about love. At the time we were constantly defining all sorts of terms and we began to see that love had as many shadings as the public library had volumes. For example, I had a crush on my friend Merle's older brother, Lou, who was a high school senior. He drove us places and made funny, sarcastic comments. He wasn't good-looking, but I was a sucker for sarcasm.

As Merle described it, I was "madly and passionately" in love with Lou. In my case that meant I was happiest when it was Merle's mother's turn to drive because she always sent Lou in her place. This was love best enjoyed at a distance, or at least from the back seat. If he had asked me for a date I wouldn't have known what to do.

That year a bunch of us were close, boys and girls. We called ourselves a family, and over the summer after ninth grade we paired off in random fashion, bumping and moving apart like molecules. I kept a journal and about every two weeks I'd record a list of quotes under the title "Romantic Standings." They never referred to the same twosomes more than once.

At the time, "love" was often too strong a word. Or too limited. I loved my friends Harold and Al, but only as friends. The boy I *really* loved was named Mel. To cut down on the confusion, Merle defined an intermediary step between like and love. She called it "loke." We didn't use it all that much, but it opened our eyes to the many levels on which you could care about a person of the opposite sex.

When we started dating on a regular basis, the concept of

love took on new meaning. We were less likely to use it for guys we saw on Saturday nights than we had been to use it to describe our fantasy romances. It was easy to love a person you didn't have much chance of getting to know. With crushes you loved first, never really got to know the person, and eventually couldn't figure out why you'd had the crush to begin with. With boyfriends, you got to know them and either came to love them or started dating someone else.

Without giving definitions any thought, I had already assumed Fran and Sid loved each other. After all, they were married, and married people loved each other, didn't they? Over the twenty years I knew them, I assumed they had the kind of relationship they wanted, cool and distant, as opposed to close and cozy. I assumed they enjoyed their constant sniping. Each of them acted impervious and tough in the face of the other's disdainful criticisms. They responded to each other's barbs in kind. Although the meanness in their voices would have hurt *me*, I assumed they each considered that the other was joking.

But, as my son's sixth-grade teacher was always saying, never assume—it makes an "ass" out of "u" and "me." Next thing I knew, they were getting a divorce and Fran was saying she'd never loved Sid to begin with. Their divorce forced me to toss out my assumptions about their relationship. What I've decided is that Fran and Sid had not been filling each other's needs. Sid could have used a little mothering, but saying so would have meant revealing a secret, sensitive, little-boy part of himself. Fran required another adult's moral support in making domestic decisions, but asking for it would have meant admitting she wasn't always the competent, together working woman. They used meanness to mask their weaknesses, unleashed barrages of criticism to hide hurt feelings, and always needed something from each other, something they could never admit to needing.

A look at their second spouses supports my revised appraisal. Fran's new husband is a take-charge kind of guy who's trained her incorrigible dog and assigned chores to her son. Sid's new wife is a nurturing type, a spontaneous hugger who speaks to him with affection in her voice. In their search for love both Fran and Sid managed to find new spouses who satisfied their needs.

Although I know it's presumptuous of me to say so, the little I know about these new spouses suggests that their needs are also being met. Sid's wife has found in him someone steady and dependable as ballast for her offbeat, energetic self. Fran's conscientious husband has discovered through her the chance to enjoy a humorous, ironic view of life. In meeting needs, these new twosomes have a lot going for them.

And that's where Fromm made his mistake. He equated need with neurotic dependency. I don't agree. The two halves of a couple can answer each other's needs without either one becoming dependent in some incapacitating way. Answering needs can be as straightforward as "you do the cooking and I'll do the yardwork," as unspoken as "you need mothering and I'm the mothering type." When the need fits with the giver's talents, no one is resentful.

I've never had the opportunity to talk to Fran about all this. I'd like to tell her my theory, which is that love and need are tightly intertwined. If you love someone, it's because he satisfies your needs on some level. By the same token, loving someone obligates you to figure out what his needs are and meet them as best you can. If you aren't willing to do that, then you probably don't love him. And if he isn't taking care of your needs, then whether or not you once loved him hardly matters.

As an aftereffect of all this, since Fran and Sid split up I've been considering what Michael would look for if he had the chance to choose another woman.

Like him, she would play a musical instrument for pleasure and, at a concert, hear the notes in a way I never can. She would know that Shostakovich can be listened to correctly only at top volume. She would learn to fly his single-engine plane instead of reading a novel in the copilot's seat. His new woman would always wake up cheerful and never have a grumpy Sunday. She wouldn't talk him into eating at Mexican restaurants, seriously suggest visiting the dog museum in St. Louis, or need the covers straightened just so before she went to sleep. She would like drifting off to John Wayne movies, crave fried liver, never want to shop.

If Michael ever read this, he would laugh. Yes, he'd like for me to become a pilot, have a more natural ear for classical music, never be crabby. But he'd also laugh because these are details. The same is true on my side. Sure, I'd like a husband who thought restaurant dining was the best way to go, considered clothes at least moderately important, didn't whistle. But this is trivia.

The reason neither of us is out looking for someone new after twenty-three years of marriage is plain and simple: We fill each other's needs. I need someone warm and cuddly and sympathetic; he's a terrific hugger and an excellent listener. He needs to see love demonstrated, and over the years, I've learned how to show him lots of affection. Inevitably, when one of us feels pessimistic, the other supplies the optimistic outlook.

This abstract list could go on, but perhaps it's enough to say that we are complementary. What one of us is missing the other supplies.

Never Confess

LAURA GREEN

Henry Ford II didn't say much about automobiles that sticks in the mind but he was elegant on the subject of infidelity. Perhaps the subject was closer to his heart than Mustangs and Thunderbirds. Maybe he was having one transcendent moment of common sense. Whatever. When his second marriage was breaking up and reporters were hounding him about rumors that he was seeing a younger woman, he had only one thing to say: "Never explain, never complain." And that was all he ever said about his relationship with the woman who became his third wife.

Henry Ford was right. Whoever said "Suffer in silence" was probably talking about extramarital relationships. He must have known there is no good way to explain an affair. Better not to discuss it at all.

Am I telling the unfaithful to be dishonest as well as disloyal? Well, yes, I guess I am. Admitting to adultery (what an old-fashioned word for such a timeless vice!) instantly makes a bad situation much worse. The admission of infidelity brings so much pain to the person hearing the confession that it can never be the right thing to do. No matter what the justification—and there will always be plenty of them—infidelity is a treacherous act. Either you don't discuss it or you do, and it changes the nature of your relationship irrevocably.

Is it time for a disclaimer? I think so. I suppose I have a double standard. Cheating is okay for other people, but not for me and my husband. As far as I am concerned, infidelity is the refuge of the desperate and I am not one of the desperate. I am a listener, though, and years ago, before I realized that it is often better not to know, I spent a decade of hearing painful stories of fragile marriages and relationships knocked flat by affairs. I learned too much about couples cracked apart by lovers. In earlier relationships, I had been cheated on and it hurt. Maybe that made me sound as if I knew more about love and forgiveness than I did. Perhaps my friends were reaching a certain stage in their lives. Whatever the reason, I attracted long, tortured confessions from betrayed—and betraying—friends.

What I learned is what Henry Ford said: Never explain, never complain. And I came to believe the unspoken corollary, too: "Never confess, never ask forgiveness." Not to friends. Not to mate. Not to anyone, ever.

For what it's worth, silence spares your friends as well as your spouse. I was once awakened at four or five in the morning by a bleary, unshaven, distraught man who demanded to know whether his wife was having an affair. Unfortunately, she was, and, worse, she had told me all about it. She had been unhappily married for years and the inevitable happened, although her story was far more complicated than my summary. Even as I was hearing my friend's confessions, I realized I was learning more than I wanted to know, particularly the part about how she and her husband rarely wanted to make love and why it was never really any good when they did. So there I was in my bathrobe as the poor man shoved his way past me into my apartment and stood there, red-eyed and exhausted. I am ashamed to say I didn't feel sorry for him. Despite his naked pain, I felt sorry for myself. I didn't know what to do or say. Lie? Tell him the truth? Shut the door in his face?

I still feel bad about what I did. I should have lied to spare him the humiliation of knowing that he knew, and to save myself from the scene that followed. But I just mumbled something to the effect that his wife was seeing another man. What can I say? I was in my mid-twenties, untouched by life and uncomfortable with any grief but my own. I was shaken by his undisguised anguish and frightened by his fury. I rationalized and believed him when he said he already knew. He said his wife had told him all about it. Maybe she had, maybe not. Maybe he knew, maybe I was the one who told him. Shortly after that, they separated, and even though I believed their marriage had been on a respirator, I sometimes wondered if I was the one who'd pulled the plug.

No matter how strained the relationship, sexual betrayal is a terrible rejection, for it rejects your most naked, vulnerable self. Nowhere do we reveal ourselves more honestly than when we make love with abandon. In uninhibited lovemaking we reach back and grab the ecstasy of infancy. Floating on desire, we know the lightheaded joy of feeling without thought. Infidelity kills all that, leaving you exposed, ashamed, self-conscious, and betrayed.

It is also an awful awakening for the one who is unfaithful. Cheating loosens the bonds you once thought could never be bent—knowledge that is rarely worth having, much less sharing. You might think that having an affair is like finally leaving Omaha, but it is really like leaving Eden because it destroys everyone's innocence. In confession's hothouse of repudiation, humiliation, and rejection it is simply not possible to say "I'm sorry" and wait for forgiveness. So why do so many men and women keep confessing?

Over the years, I have come to believe that the purpose of telling the truth is to ease the teller's burdens and mortally wound the listener, not to clear the decks and start over. The primary purpose of confessing is to make the confessor feel better, usually at the expense of the one who must forgive. That is why the Roman Catholic Church's practice of having priests hear confession was a stroke of genius. In a religion that forbids divorce, the neutral confessional is essential.

We also believe in public confession with a naive faith that cannot be shaken by reality. No matter how often we are disgusted by celebrities' admissions and neighbors' confessions, we still think it will sound better when we do it. My generation grew up convinced that talk cures everything. Get things off your chest, we say. Don't hold them in, you'll get an ulcer. We believe that unspoken grievances fester, making women overeat and men drink too much. Cursed with the predisposition to bare our souls, we babble, never asking whether the relief of admission is worth the damage it causes.

Which brings us back to the virtues of silence. Keeping your sins to yourself is not just a compassionate gesture toward someone you probably still love, it is also the keenest punishment for infidelity's pleasures. Nothing is more satisfying than boasting what a wonderful lover your lover is. Nothing puts down your mate more memorably. To refuse to gloat aloud, on the other hand, is to pass a rigorous test of will and exercise some long-overdue self-denial.

That is why the wise adulterer does not ask for forgiveness. It is too much to ask. Honest men and women know that although adultery may be justifiable, it does not follow that it also is forgivable. Knowing they are in the wrong, they shut up and get on with life. In a much, much different context, such a person is what my father would have called a mensch, a Yiddish word that translates as man but really means a stand-up guy, someone who can be relied upon to do the right thing without making a fuss over it.

Which is why you should never turn to friends for moral support, or brag about your beautiful lover, or tell your mate and beg for forgiveness. The only compassionate answer to the question "Have you slept with anyone else since we got married?" is "Of course not." Like the question "Am I a failure?", it does not seek the truth. Instead, it begs for reassurance.

If you must confess to friends, there is a proper way to do it. That was brought home to me by an unhappy friend who poured out her heart about some desperate flings as we watched our toddlers at the playground. She said that if her husband should ever confront me with questions about her lovers, I should say: "I think you had better discuss that with your wife." I was to stand firm on that point; she insisted. She would handle it. There was no need for me to go any deeper into it. I appreciated her willingness to face the music. I think now that it was her way of thanking me for listening as she tried to work it all out. (They're no longer married, either.)

The one good thing I can say for confession is that it's the quick kill, the pinpoint bombing. It is certainly more honest than creating a situation where you get yourself found out and try to provoke your partner into leaving you. I don't even want to get into stories of mislaid bills from the jeweler or the hotel.

More often, when someone approves of confession, they're not thinking of mercy killing. They're thinking of revenge for the disappointments of marriage. Even an Einstein, lost in the stars, knows that a prime reason for affairs is to settle scores. The grievances that drive someone to adultery may be varied, but one factor is always the same: the cold satisfaction of sticking it to your partner. The unlovely truth is that vengeance is very satisfying, at least as satisfying as cheating itself—and the pleasure lasts longer.

Revenge may be a dish best served cold, but there is no question that it also tastes better served in front of witnesses. It takes a person of great character to be satisfied with savoring its sweetness secretly. If only it were enough to gloat in private and let it go at that.

Nothing can make adultery as easy to accept as it is to justify. Its punishment should be never to boast to friends or grovel or beg forgiveness of a mate. Revel in secret, repent in private, suffer in silence. Having been a real jackass, your best recourse now is to become a mensch.

Material Girl

MAGDA KRANCE

I didn't know exactly what to expect on my first Mother's Day, but I did expect something.

I had, after all, been colonized by our baby for nine months. Labor had lived up to its name and then some. After a dozen hours of intense yet somehow dreamy pain that pulled me repeatedly from the edge of fitful sleep, I pushed for nearly six hours before our son emerged, battered and yowling and, as it turned out, not entirely well. Postpartum wooziness and euphoria were muddled by the anxiety of having our baby taken away to the intensive care unit. My hormones and emotions churned violently just beneath my necessarily calm, coping surface. The baby's needs came first.

He survived. We survived. And a month later, it was Mother's Day.

I don't know what I wanted, but I wanted something significant—a grand gesture, a tribute to the fact that I had just

made a baby in my body, that I had suffered while pushing
him into the world, that I had given my husband a son. We
did it together, of course, but biology made me the one who
was physically and emotionally occupied and then drained by
the experience. I felt I fully deserved to be lauded for my
effort, sacrifice, and success. This was, after all, unlike anything I'd ever done before—more basic, more significant, more
cosmic.

That's not to say I had any specific expectations—only a
pleasant, vague anticipation of something special happening.
And when nothing did, I was devastated.

The morning of Mother's Day, I woke first and wandered
into the dining room. The usual disarray of newspapers and
placemats littered the table. There was no greeting card or
gift-wrapped acknowledgment that the day was noteworthy,
no prelude to what I'd hoped would be a day of loving surprises. Disappointment pricked me. I ate the usual weekday
breakfast of cold cereal, alone. Other new mothers might be
served breakfast in bed, or taken to brunch, but not me. The
self-pity began percolating. Eventually, my husband got up
with the baby. As I read the papers, still faintly hopeful, I
heard him scribbling in his office. A few minutes later he
dropped a card on the table in front of me on his way to the
kitchen, without even stopping to hug or kiss me.

That was it. A card. Dismay and anger welled up like
lava. A card! I could scarcely read it, I was so hurt. Was that
all that having a baby was worth? Was that the thank-you I
got for what I'd gone through?

As the day went on, I felt more betrayed and bitter. The
air buzzed with his anxiety and my hurt. I was sure that
other new mothers were being treated royally by their devoted
spouses. I even felt mocked by the Sunday comics, which
were full of tender Mother's Day tributes. By the time a mes-
senger arrived some hours later with a low-budget arrange-
ment of flowers, I was nearly blind with my sense of

woundedness. Nothing could mollify me. A week earlier, we'd received a similar bouquet from a distant friend, congratulating us on our son's birth, and I'd been touched. Somehow, though, I expected more than a few carnations from my mate—a permanent memento, something that showed thought and imagination, something beyond the baldly obligatory.

Later that day, when I began crying as Steve dressed to go play soccer, as he does every weekend, his lips twisted in exasperation. "I *knew* this was going to happen!" he said, as if his failure to anticipate my expectations was somehow my fault and not a further indictment of his lack of thoughtfulness, as if I had no right to be disappointed that he'd essentially done nothing for Mother's Day. Which, of course, made me cry more.

Granted, we were both new to being parents, and Mother's Day had previously meant long-distance calls to our own mothers. Granted, the typical stresses of new parenthood had been amplified by our son's cerebral hemorrhage and the barrage of follow-up neurological examinations. Granted, my husband was distracted by the financial burden brought on by the baby's complications, and I was still overwhelmed by the myriad changes wrenching my body and psyche.

If anything, we needed to celebrate all the more because of what we'd gone through. I know I did. During pregnancy, mothers-to-be are a magnet of attention; after birth, women go through a sort of withdrawal as all eyes turn to the newborn, who is relentlessly demanding and dependent.

Confronted by my inescapable tears, Steve finally decided that it would be appropriate to do something together as a family. Without a word he changed back into street clothes and suggested we go for a walk. I wanted to be grateful, really. Instead, I felt like shattered glass. This was no minor slight. The damage was not readily repaired. I snuffled miserably as we walked, thinking of all the simple things he could have done or said, thinking how easy the day should have been, but unable to say anything without sounding accusatory and bitchy.

There is, I realize, often a chasm between the expectations of men and women where gifts are concerned. Most men seem happy with practical, dorfy things that would plunge most women into deep depression—tool kits, Weber grills, the masculine equivalents of washing machines and ironing boards. For the most part, women want gifts with emotional meaning. Simple enough. So why do so many men have gift dyslexia?

For myself and many women I know, a gift should be an expression of thoughtfulness and affection, not of mere duty. It should be wanted, but it should also surprise. Ideally, it should answer at least some of these questions: What would she love to be seen in? to read? to look at? to listen to? to feel next to her skin? What can I give her that will be for her pleasure alone, that will have nothing to do with cooking or housework or office work or furnishing the house? A gift should say, "Your happiness is important to me, so I took the time to find something you would love." A gift is a symbol.

I think women instinctively know this, while a lot of men seem not to. There are exceptions, but for the most part, men don't like to put themselves on the line by giving gifts. Maybe it's a phallic thing; they fear being rejected if their offering isn't big enough or good enough. They do it when they absolutely have to, but they're generally uncomfortable about it. Their gift-giving doesn't spring from some yearning to be loved, but from a wary sense of obligation. They have to do it. They dread and resent it. Or a lot of them do, anyway.

If my husband needs me to draw him a roadmap, then it doesn't count, because he doesn't have to put any thought into it, and there is no surprise. Ultimately, it *is* the thought that counts, which means there has to be *some* thought. If I must tell him that there's something at a certain shop that I'd really like, he's not getting a gift as much as running an errand. It brings no real joy.

I am not a whiner, generally. I am not hopelessly self-centered. I try to be thoughtful and caregiving and loving to my family and friends. I remember special occasions with gifts and cards—and I assume, I guess, that my thoughtfulness will be reciprocated.

Am I really so petty, so materialistic, to be upset when it isn't? The world is full of domestic violence, broken marriages, poverty and despair. I am unquestionably blessed. What Steve wrote in that Mother's Day card was beautiful, heartfelt, deeply moving. When I finally could read it, much later, it made me weep with gratitude and remorse.

So why wasn't that enough? He loves me, he loves me lots. He loves me, he loves me lots. "He loves me not" isn't part of the picture. I know that beyond any doubt. His love is a constant presence, sturdy and resilient and dependable.

Why isn't simple, sturdy love enough? Can't love just be, and be its own reward? Why do I expect material proof on special occasions, tangible gestures of thoughtfulness and appreciation? Why am I so devastated when none is forthcoming?

And why, after almost fourteen years together, doesn't he know that, beyond any doubt?

When he does get it right, I melt. On my birthday a few years ago, at a wonderfully splurgy four-star restaurant, he tenderly proffered a small velvety box the color of chocolate mousse. My stomach butterflied, the way it had so often when we first fell in love. Opening the little box, I gasped to find a gold band with ten small diamonds lined up like podded peas—completely unexpected. It was an early tenth-anniversary ring, he explained with a shy smile; that date was still months away. My eyes blurred with happy tears. It was a wonderful moment, one I can relive whenever I glance at that beautiful ring on my hand, as I often do.

It's not just me. I think men and women all crave such

moments. Life is largely a continuum of responsibility and routine. If we're lucky, our days and nights pass smoothly, punctuated with friendly pats and kisses, satisfying love, and the occasional bunch of flowers. Birthdays, anniversaries, Mother's Day and Father's Day, and assorted other occasions are society's way of telling the individual, "You are somebody. You are appreciated. You are important to me. We celebrate your birth, your commitment to marriage, to parenthood." Special recognition breaks up the routine. It gives us all something to work for, to look forward to. It doesn't have to be prohibitively expensive. It does have to be special, to reflect extra thought and attention.

Is that so hard to understand?

Telling

LAURIE ABRAHAM

I

As a child, I considered the advice columns of Dear Abby and Ann Landers windows into a mysterious, vaguely sinister adult world of love and lust, loneliness and heartbreak, divorce and betrayal. I read the columns avidly, marveling at the fixes adults got themselves into and nodding in agreement with the level-headed advice Abby and Ann dished out. The two columnists were like reliable big sisters; they wouldn't steer you wrong. That's why I was amazed one day to read Abby, or maybe it was Ann, advising "Guilty" *not* to tell her husband about her short-lived fling with another man. If the affair was

truly an aberration, Abby counseled, then no good could be
served by telling all. The woman would only hurt her husband by telling, Abby said. What? Abby advocated concealing
an affair? I was shocked. When my mother had told me never
to tell a lie, I had not only obeyed her, I had believed that it
was a rule adults followed, too. The only ones who did otherwise, at least that I knew of, were the well-coiffed, bejeweled
seductresses who preened through the soap operas my mother
and I watched while she ironed. I assumed that my experiences would never approach theirs, with or without an emer-
ald cocktail ring on my finger.

I stored away the baffling bit of advice, but as I progressed
through high school, then college, I began to quote it as gos-
pel. It is silly and indulgent to confess to small affairs, I would
say to my friends when they debated whether or not to tell.
I advised them to examine their motives. Were they telling
just to relieve their own guilt, or perhaps to wound an inatten-
tive lover? The confession of fleeting sexual transgressions,
and the uncompromising standard of honesty that demanded
it, seemed foolish, if not selfish. I remembered a friend who
had opened his message to me in my ninth-grade yearbook
with "Other people may not like you, but I do." His statement
was undoubtedly true (though I still wonder who he was talking about), but such "honesty" was obviously misguided. His
comment had devastated my tender fifteen-year-old psyche,
and from a distance, it seems akin to blabbing about a meaningless affair.

My first and only affair, if you could call it that, confirmed
my theory. I was twenty-two and in the fourth year of my
first serious relationship, with a boy I had met in high school.
It was the summer after I graduated from college, and we
were living together in Chicago. Once or twice a week, I
worked the night shift at the newspaper where I was interning
and took the train home afterward. On one of these evenings,
a blond, curly-haired lawyer whom I had met while wait-

ressing at a wedding reception tapped my shoulder and rein-
troduced himself. The funny thing was that I was sitting next
to a man who a few minutes earlier had approached me on
the train, a man I knew in passing from college but who now
seemed intent on knowing me better. Here I was, bleary-eyed
and disheveled after typing police stories and obituaries onto
a glowing green computer screen until 11 p.m., and two men
were eagerly vying for my attentions. It felt great.

    In the end, with the train nearing my stop, I opted for
attorney Jay because he had better hair and flattered me more
shamelessly. He was also more forceful. He grabbed my arm
as we got off the train and looked into my eyes, insisting that
I accompany him to a nearby bar for a drink. Warmed by a
carafe of red wine, we talked nonstop, leaning toward each
other across a red-and-white gingham table cloth, our eyes
reflecting candlelight. At about 1:30, he asked me if I would
meet him the next night for dinner. I nervously agreed and
walked the couple of blocks home to my boyfriend. Paul was
asleep, so I undressed and climbed into bed with him. He
mumbled something about my whereabouts, and I told him
I'd been drinking with some friends after work. I felt slightly
guilty about my lie but was still dazed by my newfound desir-
ability. And Paul and I had been having problems. I quickly
fell asleep.

    I did meet Jay for dinner: fettuccine alfredo served at his
apartment, it turned out. We both got drunk once again, went
to a bar and got drunker, then came back to his apartment
and had sex. I would have preferred not to, but it seemed to
be what was expected after our whirlwind two nights. It was
not a case of what has come to be known as date rape. The
whole fling had been an adventure for me, and sex was the obvious
culmination of it. The day after, I remembered the act only
dimly, but I knew I had not liked it, that Jay had been (surprise!) aggressive and rather crude. I was about to leave for
Washington, D.C., for another newspaper internship, and de-

cided not to see him again. It would have been absurd to tell
Paul about this incident: "Paul, I need to tell you I had ugly
sex with a man I met on the 'el' train, and I never want to
see him again. I just thought you should know." It seemed
even more absurd to confess the incident after I ran into Jay
several months later. "Hi, Babe, how ya doin'?" he said. He
sounded like a lounge singer in a nearly empty hotel bar. His
hair looked brassy in the noon light, and red lines spidered
the whites of his eyes. Thank God I didn't tell Paul, I thought
to myself. Seeing Jay in this new light, I imagined what I
might have told Paul now: "Paul, I need to tell you I had ugly
sex with a man who talks like Bill Murray imitating a washed-
up nightclub performer. I never want to see him again. I just
thought you should know."

II

Approaching affairs from the other side, that of the potentially
cheated-upon girlfriend, I do not behave like a woman who
believes that telling, and the knowing that inevitably accompanies it, is dangerous and needlessly painful. It's embarrassing
to admit, but I've riffled through my current boyfriend's
address book, twitching with the desire to ring up all the
women whose names I do not recognize. I even called one
once but hung up as soon as someone answered. What
would I have said? "My boyfriend asked me to clean out
his address book. Do you still merit a listing?" Mike has
never given me reason to suspect him of infidelity. I've con-
ducted these searches when I'm alone and I spot the black
book sitting invitingly on the buffet or calling to me from
an open drawer. My thoughts hurtle off into a dark world
of mistrust and deception, and suddenly I'm sure that Mike
must be having a torrid affair.

My demented curiosity is partly the product of the distance between Mike and me. For two years now, we have

spent nine months of the year apart while he attends school in a town a thousand miles away. I can't help wondering what goes on after one of the law school's parties. Does Mike sneak a kiss with an East Coast girl who wears simple but obscenely expensive clothes and comes from a good family? I have tried to figure out why I can be overcome by a powerful urge to know when I believe that knowing could wreak unnecessary havoc on my relationship. The best answer I can come up with is that rational-thinking people can act in self-destructive ways.

I've mulled over the possibility that learning Mike had a fling wouldn't bother me as much as I imagine, but I doubt I could ever be satisfied that a fling was *only* that and nothing more. The idea of my lover sleeping with another woman could not be laughed off or forgotten. I could not escape the suspicion that the affair was a harbinger of doom, a sign that his love for me was flagging. Nothing he could say would lessen my fear of abandonment, my sense of inadequacy. He might swear that she meant nothing to him, that it's over, that she was the result of too many martinis and too many lonely nights without me—the woman he really loves—but none of that would comfort me. I would still hate him. No amount of protesting could eliminate the revulsion I would feel when I imagined him in bed with another woman.

Dear Abby was right. It's best not to know—or tell.

Temptation

JANICE ROSENBERG

Here's the setup.

A couple of weeks ago my nephew (I'll call him Ben) was in town for a job interview. Ben is twenty-seven years old and single. A friend of his from graduate school out East (I'll call her Marcy) helped arrange the job interview at the Chicago company where she works.

I assumed that Marcy was single. Ben had recently broken up with his girlfriend, and I wondered idly whether there was any possibility for romance with Marcy. Ben stayed with Marcy on Sunday night and Monday night. On Tuesday he had his interview and came to our house, where he stayed for two nights.

Ben is charming and intelligent. We had a nice, chatty visit. When he mentioned that Marcy had a husband, I was more disappointed than surprised. Ben's stay with her had nothing to do with scouting out a new girlfriend. In fact, Ben and Marcy were never romantically involved. They were, and are, as the saying goes, just friends.

Ben knows Marcy's husband, too. He's still a graduate student on the East Coast. He commutes to Chicago on weekends and therefore wasn't present during Ben's stay.

My husband gave me this last bit of information the day after Ben went home, in what could only be called a tone of

restrained moral outrage. Ben and Marcy had been alone together in her apartment for two consecutive nights, he said. I
could feel him waiting for my response, already guessing his
opinion—that staying unchaperoned with a married woman
was a very bad idea.

No similar alarms went off in my head. Their two nights
sounded perfectly innocuous to me, comparable in style with
their college lives in coed dorms and off campus male-female
shared apartments. Michael and I had no firsthand knowledge
of those kinds of living arrangements. Maybe if he had, he'd
be less dogmatic. Or, a little voice said, maybe he'd be more
so.

I sighed silently and prepared to state my case. I knew
from the outset that I would be backed into an untenable
position. In all our arguments on subjects like this I take the
most liberal view to counteract what I see as his puritanical
one. He has no trouble being absolutist. I'm the one whose
argument always disintegrates because I see too many shades
of gray.

So I said that I thought it was okay for Ben to stay with
Marcy. They were just friends. Men and women could be
just friends. Although I had no recent experience to back up
my statement, in high school I had enjoyed numerous male
friendships of the not-romantically-inclined variety. I could
empathize with Ben and Marcy. They enjoyed each other's
company, but they weren't attracted to each other in the usual
boy-girl way.

Michael didn't accept that premise. He understands the
concept of male-female friendship, but he believes strongly
that there is an element of sexual attraction in every such
relationship simply because sexual attraction is an intrinsic
part of what draws men and women together as friends. For
him, the two ways of relating—as friends and sexually—are
inseparable.

This doesn't mean he thinks men and women can never

be together without sexuality getting in the way. Sure, men and women work in offices together, meet as halves of couples, interact in organizations of all sorts. What he means is that an effort must be made at all times by those who are not available for romance—i.e., married people—to repress that sexual awareness, to keep it in check. How do you do that? Well, first of all, by avoiding situations that foster sexuality.

For Michael the rules are straightforward. Marriage means being faithful and being faithful does not include flirtation, surreptitious eye contact, little touches, or evenings spent alone with people of the opposite sex. Human beings, he thinks, are basically weak. They should not put themselves in the way of temptation. Therefore, no matter what Ben and Marcy *said* they felt about each other, they should not have been together overnight at Marcy's apartment while her husband was away.

If you liked the person enough to spend an evening with him or her, Michael said, it was a too-short step from sipping wine on the couch to the look that says okay, why not? What's wrong with a little experimenting? It won't mean that I don't love my spouse. It won't mean anything.

He paused, having stated his argument, and it was my turn. People weren't that weak, I said. Or if they were that weak, or so inclined, they didn't need the opportunity of a spouse out of town for the inevitable to happen. A person who would seduce or allow him- or herself to be seduced by an overnight guest was already a time bomb waiting to explode. His or her marriage was unsteady to begin with. If, on the other hand, you had decided that you would be faithful to your spouse, you built a fence that protected you from temptation. A friend could spend the night at your apartment and nothing would happen.

Michael built his fence further back. He said that the only way to avoid temptation was for married people to remove themselves completely from all situations that might involve it. That meant not being alone with a so-called friend of the opposite sex where there were no obstacles to keep you from following your romantic inclinations. Because married people, like any other kind of people, couldn't help having them. They had them and they couldn't completely repress them. They shouldn't even try. Sexuality was part of human nature. A lifetime of monogamy was a lot to expect and probably not at all natural. But it was the way our society had evolved, and if you signed on, you were supposed to stick to it.

Michael had another point to make. Temptation didn't have to evolve into sexual activity for the event to be disturbing to the left-out spouse. Jealousy doesn't need reality to feed it. Even if there was not the slightest, tiniest hint that anything physical had happened between Ben and Marcy, her husband might still wonder what they'd done after lights out. He was likely to feel hurt that while he was away studying, his wife and another man had enjoyed a pleasant couple of evenings going to dinner and chatting about old times. He might be troubled by her need for an evening of any kind with another man. He might feel foolish about his feelings, but he would feel them anyway. Would he be able to tell Marcy that he wasn't happy allowing her the kind of freedom young couples supposedly allow each other nowadays? A lot depended on the balance of their relationship. Which of them had more power? Which loved or needed the other more? How had they arranged their commuter marriage? Had either any reason not to trust the other?

Listening, I knew that Michael was attributing his own feelings and insecurities to Marcy's spouse. He was telling me, without saying in so many words, how he would feel if I allowed a male friend to spend the night while he was out of town. And I could tell that this spending-the-night scenario was less something he thought might happen than a symbol for all kinds of tempting male-female possibilities that I could

become involved in as, clearly, I thought male-female friendships were okay.

As our discussion moved forward, I knew we were no
longer talking strictly about Ben and Marcy, or even about
Michael and me. The two of them began to stand for any
man and any woman. How I felt about Ben and Marcy had
to be tested for its usefulness as a categorical imperative. In
other words, did my view that their sleeping arrangements
were okay apply in every situation? For example, what if Ben
and Marcy *had* once been romantically involved? Or what if,
unknown to one of them, the other had a major crush on him
or her? Or what if, God forbid, the guy turned out to be
a date-rapist? Or the woman, just to be fair, some kind of
seductress?

I didn't want to back off because I so much *want* men and
women to be able to be friends. At the same time I am familiar
with the certain sexual awareness that I have from time to
time with other men. Just last spring there was this man we
met on our vacation in the Bahamas. . . . Nothing happened.
But I could see that he was a man I'd enjoy flirting with if I
allowed myself that luxury. I was pleased to see that Michael
liked his wife. While they talked about their childhoods in
New York, the man and I had the tiniest flirtation cloaked in
meaningless conversation. It wasn't even a flirtation. It was a
flirtation with flirtation, my fence being firmly in place. Distant as it was from the real thing, I enjoyed the sensation, felt
good to know that I could still attract another man if I wanted
to.

So I know what Michael's talking about. And I don't really
believe that it's always okay for men and women to do what
Ben and Marcy did.

What I really think is that it's okay for a friend of the
opposite sex to spend the night alone with you if you have
absolutely no intention of being anything but completely faithful to your spouse. The problem is in knowing whether you

have that intention. There are so many layers of human desire.
You can say to yourself, I plan to remain completely faithful
to my spouse. We have a good relationship, communicate
well, have a great sex life. Why would I want to sleep with
someone else?

In my argument with Michael I said more than once that
if you were in a position to step out of the bounds of marriage,
you will find a way to do it. Having a friend stay over just
makes it easy. My husband said, why make it easy? I said, if
you aren't predisposed to doing it, you won't. That was the
crux of the matter. He feels we're all always predisposed and
should stay out of danger. I feel that I can make the decision
in a rational way. He thinks you can be drawn in despite your
best and strongest rational willpower.

A week later we spent an evening with Ben's brother. He
has been married for two years and we asked him and his
wife what they thought of Ben's overnight. They said Ben
and Marcy were definitely just friends with no prior romantic
relationship. We asked, how would you feel? They said, well
if it were an old boy- or girlfriend, then yes, they wouldn't
like it. But if it were a friend—and they named several, testing
each other—then it would be okay.

They put a practical spin on the argument. Why tell a
friend to spend money on a hotel when he can stay with you
for free? But Ben, my husband pointed out, could have stayed
all four nights with us. Or the company where he was inter-
viewing would have paid for his stay at a nice downtown
hotel. He could have visited with his friend, said good-night,
and instead of merely closing the guest-room door, gone off
to sleep at a safer distance.

The argument, of course, can never be resolved. Every
case is different. None of us can tell when we'll suddenly
be attracted to someone toward whom we previously felt no
romantic urge. It could be the lamplight, the music, a sudden

loneliness, a recent fight you had with your spouse. It could be simple curiosity or the other person's loneliness.

I scoffed at this. Aren't we all old enough to control our animal urges? My husband says he's not, and holds that rule out for everyone. Trust has nothing at all to do with it. People are weak. Sexuality is strong. Why take the chance?

Months later, I continue to feel frustrated by his narrow view of male-female relationships. I don't want to believe that there is no such thing as platonic friendship, that, like Harry and Sally, we are all destined one day to succumb. I tell myself there can be satisfying conversations, friendly lunches, telephone chats that lead to nothing more. At the same time I know the possibility of getting physical sizzles to some extent below the surface of every male-female friendship. We would enjoy our friendships so much less if that weren't true.

Touchy

LAURA GREEN

One night last spring on the way home from the movies, I began to cry. It was probably the first time in a decade I had started crying without understanding why. I usually know the reason for my tears, and I am of the opinion that a good cry is as comforting and homey as a cup of tea. But that night, when my husband asked me what was wrong, I had no idea.

I do know this, though. It doesn't take much to make me cry and it doesn't take much to make me angry.

My husband and I have two different explanations for this, which we discuss late at night in clipped tones. Sometimes when we are done, I roll over and put my arm around him and we fall asleep together. Sometimes I think, "I can't possibly sleep in the same bed as this man," and go off to another bedroom.

For years my explanation has been that I am weary of the chores of marriage—who isn't? My husband and I have been together nearly twenty years and the work hasn't let up. Nor has his refusal to accept that half of it is his. I won't bore you with the details save to say that there are a lot of them. Neither of us has enough free time, but I will go to my grave thinking I did the lion's share (not to mention the lioness's). I am tried of being the generalissimo of household jobs. He is tired of hearing about it. When I am buried, my husband will put up a stone that says, "She finally gave it a rest."

My husband's explanation is much simpler: hormones. You are getting near menopause, he tells me. You are not yourself these days. No matter what he says or how he says it, I hear condescension in his voice. That's when I fold my arms and glower and declare that I am too tough-minded to get depressed by such things. But look at your friend, he says, she's a lot tougher than you are and she got so tired of slamming her office door so she could cry that she is now on estrogen. On some level, my husband thinks that women are not fully rational and living with a perimenopausal woman has given him ammunition for a lifetime's worth of argument on this point. I'll be damned if I'll add to it, though in my heart I know he is at least as right as I am.

I suspect it has to do with needing order at this point in my life, but in our household, hormones brought the issues of housework to a nasty head. I ran out of patience over the stuff that nobody but I did and I went on a yearlong tirade. I became incapable of discussing the laundry or the wet towels on the couch without exploding. Our vehement arguments over domestic issues sometimes drove me to our cold little spare-room bed where even my beloved dog, snoring softly on my feet, couldn't warm my stony heart. My husband was upstairs in our bedroom, rigid but asleep. I was in another bedroom downstairs, crying into a pillow.

I can't blame it all on hormones.

I have been furious with him over both the housekeeping chores and the family chores since the first diaper needed changing. We have had these blowups for years, usually ending with my accusation that he has no respect for women or the work that goes into raising a family and running a household. The only thing that changed about our arguments is that a few years ago, I stopped apologizing when I was done yelling. I kept on yelling. I was so angry at what I saw as my family's refusal to take responsibility for themselves that I declared war on the people I loved, especially my husband.

My fury lasted about a year and it effected a turnaround that redistributed the workload. For it, I paid a price. There were many nights when I was the pariah, palpably unwelcome when I walked into the room where my husband, son, and daughter sat. No one liked me much, especially me, but I battled my way toward a more equitable life with some time for myself in it. Other people have learned to catch flies with honey. It is my lot in life to smash them flat.

We rarely argued over big things. That would have been like setting the house afire. The big things rarely do you in, though they run like a subterranean river, numbing the heart. They cause resentment but they do not go unresolved. You buy a house or you don't. You have another baby or you don't. You move across the country or you stay put. You stay married or you separate. It's the indignities that are safe to fight over, the little abdications on his part, or the wisecracks on mine that say, I don't respect you.

Our frictions rub us raw because we are so different. We are an odd couple, compatible in our values but inept at exer-

cising them on a day-to-day basis. We both can rise to the
occasion, handling crises well. We'd be good people to have
around during a flood. It's the steady rain of ordinary life that
we can't handle, the routine of mess, dishes, bills, repairmen,
and responsibilities, responsibilities, responsibilities.

I am ready to blame my quick anger on impending menopause. But that's only a fantasy. There is no end point to our
squabbling, no day after which we will have only rational,
calm disputes. No, we fight because of who we are. Because
of who I am. Because I see slights in every gesture.

I am so touchy because we are so close to what I believe
our marriage can be despite our chronic disharmony. So close.
The children are growing up. Our daughter is about to leave
for college and our son is entering high school. This is the
last mile of the marathon. In a year or two we will have the
time together that we need. If only I don't blow it in my
anger and say something I can never take back.

Over time in a marriage, the highs make up for the lows
in a cycle of anger, reconciliation, forgiveness, understanding,
consideration, forgetfulness, and hurt. Our lives have see-
sawed from the light to the shadow, rocking like boats at
their moorings, looking for homeostasis. Our up years have
balanced the down ones. But we have just come out of a year
when I nearly tipped us over. That's what frightens me, the
fear that I will sink us a few minutes before the storm finally
subsides.

Touchy is exhausting. Whether it is hormones or impatience or a desire for fairness or a longing to slough off this
stage of marriage and grow into the next, I do not know. I
do know that I am so desperate to change that I burst into
tears on the way home from the movies. A new life is there
for us and I cannot wait much longer.

The List

One of the nice things about reaching some approximation of maturity is being able to think back with a connoisseur's appreciation of your own sexual history.

When I was twenty-six and my first marriage had ended with hardly a whimper, I took on a high-profile, decently paid newspaper job in Philadelphia. I had entered my marriage as a woman who had rebelled in small ways but who still craved the approval that came from being a good girl. The two-year period before my marriage had been eventful. My mother died, which almost killed me. The first man I loved in an all-encompassing, obsessive way rejected me. I had been in a fire and suffered third-degree burns on twenty percent of my body. Although I was lucky—I survived and the fire missed my face—my arms, back, and chest were scarred. Recovery from burns is a slow, painful process and during most of the recuperation I was unable to work. Under the circumstances, I did what seemed the only sensible thing to do: I married the next man who crossed my path. Although he was sweet, it was not a marriage made in heaven. I had a son and within six months of his birth was divorced.

But now, things had changed. I had a meaningful job on a big-city newspaper. I was single again, and for some complicated reasons related to the extreme circumstances of my life before and during the marriage, I had completely lost my fear—of everything. And the women's movement had come along. The world I entered as a divorced woman was altogether new. And so was I.

The pill had been introduced in 1960. But the revolutionary notion that sex did not have to be linked to reproduction didn't connect in a big way until feminists legitimized the idea a few years later. When I was single the second time I caught a wave of the movement I would have missed if I had stayed married, and I decided to become what I'd always wanted to be: an unconventional woman. In some way I suppose that meant being a bad girl, since at the place and time where I grew up being different and being bad seemed synonymous. But good girl or bad, I made some decisions: I would become skilled at being a newspaperwoman and be successful. I would raise my son well, alone if necessary, until I married a man who would be a good father for him. I would buy some fabulous clothes to wear in my new life. And in a declaration right out of *Cosmo*, I would date the most powerful men, the most eligible bachelors in town.

First things first. The day I drew money out of my savings account to cover my apartment in Philadelphia's Rittenhouse Square, I also took out money for a new wardrobe. I drove from Connecticut to my new home city, with my household goods making the journey in a moving van. On the way to my new life, I stopped at Loehmann's and bought more good clothes than I'd ever imagined buying at one time—like a red wool pants suit, a short black dress by Bill Blass, and some cashmere sweaters and pants with pleats. Wearing pants to work (with jewelry and high heels) made a statement back then; until the day I wore pants at The *Hartford Times*, no one had ever dared. I took my bravado, my infant son, and my new wardrobe to a new city and job.

The world of newspapers, with its atmosphere of "God is on our side," was the place to be in the late sixties and early seventies. The work was exciting, the people fascinating. For the first time in my life I felt grown up and in control.

One day, the urban affairs reporter, a wise guy who had an eye that crossed unpredictably, a terrible complexion, and confidence to burn, came in and sat down in my office. He carefully closed the door behind him and said he'd heard I was a former flight attendant (or stewardess, as we were called in those years), which was his shorthand for saying I'd been a ditzy girl who couldn't possibly now be a responsible newspaper manager. It couldn't be true, could it? he asked. I remember taking a deep breath and leaning across the desk toward him. That was the old me, the nice girl, I said. The new me was a real bitch. The story was told and retold, though slightly distorted by the time it got back to me. I would never have called myself the four-letter word he used, but I didn't mind his hyperbole. Those were exaggerated days.

A couple of years later, a female reporter heard about the list of men I was keeping and told me with some rancor that I was nothing more than a power fucker. I laughed. The term didn't fit my new self-definition as a feminist, but I didn't offer a word of apology. I knew it wasn't my sex life that made her mad. If my men had been middle-class—a reporter here, a photographer there—it wouldn't have offended her so. It was the men I was choosing to conduct my sex life with that did it.

I was twenty-seven or twenty-eight, smart and blond and meeting a lot of men. I wanted to play the field on a major scale. I was learning to be unembarrassed about my pleasures. By that time I'd decided I could live a life of achievement, and observing at close range how it was done seemed like perfect training. I felt free to have relationships with whichever men I wanted. I felt free to have sexual relationships with whichever men I craved.

I organized my sex life as if I were a casting director looking for a chorus line of smart, powerful men. Later, when I had married the man I would spend the rest of my life with, he thrilled me when he said I had an unerring instinct for the most powerful man in the room. It put him in good company, I suppose, which is why he didn't object. I hadn't quite admitted it, but I thought success was sexy. In fact, my list was not about sex at all. It was about my attempt to be powerful myself.

All my life I struggled with the notion of what defined a good girl and what it meant to be unconventional and different. Old pals from high school and college remember me as adventurous. I recall being scared. What being good looked like to me then was conformity and self-sacrifice. Before feminism came along, we had so little stake in our own lives that men not only defined us, they defined how, where, and why we would live. I wanted to live my life rather than marry it. For years I had seen women falling for the wrong men as if rejection were some badge of honor, and during my own first big sexual experience I'd been so madly in love with a scoundrel and so out of control that I'd vowed I'd never let that happen again.

Now, there was a lot going on in my head. I was a girl from a small town yearning for experience. I was far less motivated by lust than curiosity. Seeing men undressed was . . . well, nice. Seeing them exercise power in their worlds was absolutely fascinating. One of my men was a politician, blessed with no insight and as randy as any of today's politicians in the news. He was also an Olympic medalist, a successful businessman, and president of an influential sports organization. Another was an academic and cabinet adviser, an important man in his field. Then there was a successful banker, not rich (I learned during those years about the rich, the super-rich, and why even highly paid wage-slaves seldom reach the last level) but possessed of great taste, civility, and a lusty persona hidden behind his banker's grays. These were worlds I wanted to know about. Like a sponge, I soaked it all up.

Then too, sexual approval can feel very satisfying for a woman, a good substitute for sexual satisfaction. I have found satisfaction in my marriage. But I needed the feelings of approval I got from the men in my life when I was in my twenties. Being openly sexual was scary, but that made it all the more delicious. I just stopped worrying about my reputation and did what I wanted to do. I suppose it was also a way to put an exclamation mark on my separation from organized religion, which had always offended me. (Later still, I would name my daughter Eve to thumb my nose at the creation myth, but that's another story.)

That list of men, indeed those years, are among my favorite memories. I learned a great deal about the role money and power play in shaping personalities—including my own.

One of my men was very rich (inherited wealth) but so modest about it that I never knew he'd gone to Exeter and Harvard (Boston, he said, when asked where he'd gone to school) until the editor of the paper where I worked, a laughably obvious social climber, told me I'd made a great catch. Didn't he see that wasn't the point? I was collecting experience. If men wanted beauty, why couldn't we women look for something that would enrich our lives, like success or sophistication or power or a good time? In the new world I was creating, *all* the men were rich or powerful. John and I never discussed his money or famous family name, and since he later decided he preferred men to women, it didn't matter. In the meantime, he designed buildings and was a sweet lover who used to pull me into doorways for long, ardent kisses as we walked back to his apartment. He was one of those excellent students who loved and retained knowledge—one of the best-educated, most confident men I've ever known.

Then there was James, the brother of the movie star who married the prince, who told funny, cynical stories about his

sister. He was tall and broad-shouldered and athletic and a
gentle lover who owned the city where he was in politics. He
took me to back-room meetings that opened my eyes to deal-
making. He was not as dumb as people said he was. I loved
having him as a notch in my belt, and when I recently returned to Philadelphia and saw East River Road changed to
his family name, I have to admit I liked it even more.

There was also the professor at the local Ivy League university who had competed with his father and was said to
have been the youngest department chairman ever. Now in
his middle forties, twenty years older than I, he took me to
parties where I was too independent to be considered a tootsie,
but too young to be for real. No one could quite figure us out.
I sat back and watched everyone compete for his attention. He
told droll stories about how they vied for his approval and
how he doled it out in dribs and drabs. A cabinet adviser, he
was approached, while we were dating, to be the president of
Berkeley. Among other things, he introduced me to the idea
that you could put someone inept in charge when you wanted
nothing to get accomplished—a power trick I have often
watched unfold in the years since then. I tried to get him to
smoke dope, but he wouldn't have anything to do with it.
Still, I think I relaxed him.

There was also, for a while, a columnist who was my first
affable cynic (a role the Irish newspaperman is uniquely suited
to), who surprised himself by falling in love with me. He was
by far the best lover of the lot, but terrible marriage material,
since in typical journalistic style he had a short attention span
and no real interest in being a husband or father. I liked him
a lot and gleefully added him to my list.

There were others. How could I forget the delicious
French banker who confided that since he wasn't an American
citizen, he was no threat to the bank president and thus would
be a safe number-two man forever? This was difficult for him,
he said; he wanted to marry a woman who stayed home all

day just panting for him to return from work, a hope that was
not too realistic in an era when women were feeling their oats.
But he was sexual to his fingertips.

In a peripheral way, this two-year period in my late twenties is about the men. But mainly they were props in an elaborate piece of theater I was playing out. In the way that
everything men and women do in their twenties is a fairly
direct response to childhood circumstances, I was evening an
old score. My mother had been completely uneducated, supporting herself and her two children as a waitress when she
met my father. According to legend, he was part of a rich
and powerful family. His family, supposedly, never approved
of the marriage. My mother, who was strong and smart and
incredibly determined, carried the pain of their disapproval to
her grave. In reality, I never once witnessed unkindness
toward my mother. My cousins are nice, middle-class men
and women who are fighting their own demons. But then, to
my mother anyway, that distance between working-class and
upper-middle-class had been an unbridgeable chasm. My interest in upper-class power and money had been my way of
thumbing my nose at the family that made her, and by exten-
sion me, feel like an outsider. Of course, if anyone had suggested that my feelings about my family were the motivation
behind having a glittering sex life, I would have laughed.
Twenty years later, I understand how I internalized my mother's anger. Wealth and power? I'd show them wealth and
power.

As the number of notches in my belt increased, so did my
confidence. I learned that sex is a good part of some relationships and not of others and that nothing can alter basic chemistry. Somewhere along the way I stopped feeling the overwhelming
need to have a man at my side. I also got tired of spending
so much time on . . . maintenance. Thinking about the right
clothes for all those occasions and keeping up my hair and

makeup and having to concentrate on looking good seemed
terribly trivial and time-consuming, as they still do.

I began to realize that I was having a lot of mediocre sex
with people I didn't really care about. I had never wanted to
be like men, playing some game where the rush of conquest
became more important than the process of love and intimacy.
And then I was right back where I'd started, believing that
sex with affection and love is best. A friend reminded me to
"call them all darling." I laughed at this advice, with its
implication that I was engaging in such great mindless sex
that I might forget their names in the heat of the moment.
But this was not great sex. Married sex, with love and leisure time, would be the transcendent experience everyone
craves.

In the meantime, my good sense rescued me and I met a
man who made my heart beat faster and who understood my
roots and who made me laugh. I knew he would be a good
father for my young son, as indeed he has been. I married
him thinking it was the end of my sexual history, when it fact
it was the beginning.

Whereas I am still glad I have a sexual history ("a woman
with a past!"), I am not so proud of the motives I had in
accumulating it. I know that the cheapest way to feel powerful
is to feel superior to others. I was indulging in the oldest game
in the world and trading sex for access. But it was the first
intentionally self-centered act in my life, and in that sense it
was the right thing to do. I want to make it clear that I was
not *giving* sex. I was taking it for myself.

The experience taught me some difficult lessons about life.
The predominant memory of my power harem is that not one
of them would have made a good husband. It takes an enormous ego to go after and retain what they had. Most powerful
men can't get out of themselves enough to consider marriage
or parenthood a genuinely important component of their lives.
It simply didn't interest them as much as it did me. I wanted

a good father for my son, and I wanted more children and a normal domestic life as well as a career. These men wanted an accessory, which today might mean smart, attractive "trophy" wives. Then, it just meant accessory.

In the long run, I believe men need women, probably more than women need men. A recent Canadian study reported that women test happier than men. Of course. We build our lives around relationships. Perhaps because of our capacity for maternity, we are softer and we think more about motivation and what constitutes contentment. We aren't as power-obsessed. Because women have had to reinvent themselves in this century, we have had to think deeply about what we want and whether the prices we'll have to pay are worth it. Younger women are better at this than women my age.

As for sexual cockiness, some of mine was faked but another part became real in the process. The old me had been afraid, so the new me had to be fearless. And where else could I have looked for power in those days, when only men had it? I also know that what Mary Wollstonecraft wrote in 1792 is just as true today as it was 200 years ago. ". . . One reason why men have . . . more fortitude than women is undoubtedly this, that they give freer scope to the grand passions and by more frequently going astray enlarge their minds."

Female virtue was invented by men, and I'm glad I went astray from the old, conventional sexual standards. By doing so, I allowed myself to make a grab for everything I wanted. Moralists would want me to confess that the entire experience was soulless and unsatisfying and that it left me feeling guilty or ashamed. They would be wrong. The fact that I changed my mind in the end has nothing to do with the beginning. I wanted to be sexual in a spontaneous, optimistic way—in other words, to express who I was in my newfound sexuality—and I did. The sex didn't make me feel loved, but it was far from anonymous. It wasn't *about* love. It was about power and independence and the freedom to make my own choices.

Over the years my feelings about status and power and love and sex have changed, although I still laugh when I think about those days and about my list. I have developed a confidence deeper than the bravado that motivated the list. My husband is the same man I met in 1970. He has an innate sense of self-worth and power. Although we are not rich or famous, he has been a wonderful father and a good husband.

BOUNDARIES

A Bedpost Without Notches

LAURIE ABRAHAM

My lover and I drove past a field of lush, green grass in Madison, Wisconsin, and he told me that that was where he and his college friends had spent lazy summer afternoons sending Frisbees soaring through the azure sky. This was during the late 1970s when his glossy brown hair flew out behind him when he ran, fell past his shoulders when he was still, when his hair took a good long time to pull your fingers through. I didn't know him then, but I've seen pictures . . . and I've imagined. Onto this field one day came a woman wearing a black leotard, tights, and a full magenta skirt. She walked deliberately, in the way that dancers do, and noticing, I suppose, the way Mike's damp hair clings to his neck after Frisbee in the sun, she asked him to rub her back. So they went to her place, to her sagging screened-in porch, and she pulled her shirt over her head and lay down on her stomach. Mike put his hands on her shoulders, and later, inevitably, they made love.

They repeated this dance several times that summer. Then she left for California, and he stayed in the Midwest to finish his philosophy degree. Today, Mike can remember that she

was an "older woman"—twenty-seven or so—who lived in a
shabby Victorian house and bathed in a claw-footed tub. What
he cannot recall, he told me, is her name. Come on, I coaxed,
you must remember; you made love to her half a dozen times.
He thought for a while, and said it might have been Nancy,
but he really was not sure.

I cannot imagine not being sure. "Rob, Paul, Jay, Mike."
My sexual roll call is on the tip of my tongue, in chronological
order, no less. To remember my lovers is as easy as counting
to four. For Mike, it's as easy as counting to twelve in a
foreign tongue, or maybe thirteen; oh yeah, fourteen, there
was that Swedish girl on the boat between London and the
Netherlands. My lack of sexual experience is a source of some
consternation to me: I've a bedpost without notches, a black
book without numbers. I have women friends who, like Mike,
take minutes as opposed to seconds to comb through their
sexual histories, pausing every once in a while with comments
like, "I know I'm forgetting someone from graduate school."
One of my dearest friends slept with twelve different men her
senior year at college. I was impressed.

I enjoy sex. I've had it regularly and joyfully with the two
men with whom I've had long-term relationships. The other
two names on my sexual log can be attributed to alcohol;
unfortunately, or perhaps not, I barely remember what happened. But despite the pleasure sex gives me, I do not spend
much time ogling random men on the street, or fantasizing
about how they might look or act in more intimate settings.
I make love in my dreams, but almost never have I "cheated
on" whomever I was making love to during my waking hours.
In general, women do less free-association fucking than men,
I know, but I believe I do less than many other women. I
suppose I've suppressed that part of me.

I've pondered the reasons for my relatively low body
count. The easiest answer is that I spent seven years in a
relationship with one man. But it's not as simple as that. For

at least a third of those seven years, my boyfriend and I lived apart, and our commitment was never ironclad. We were both young, still in college, and I had ample opportunity to experiment. Yet I let that relationship wrap me in a cocoon from which I resisted emerging for reasons that seem too mundane to mention: fear of rejection, doubt about my attractiveness to other men. These insecurities began in grade school, or perhaps junior high, where I took pride in writing the best English themes and practicing basketball with the boys but became increasingly dismayed to find that, off the court, those same boys snapped my best friend's bra strap more than mine. (It is strange to remember how chosen I felt when a boy's hand brushed my back, fumbling to snap or unhook my bra through a thin blouse.) In short, I was more adept at competing with boys—later, men—than seducing them. Taking the long view, I am thankful that my brain and athleticism were irrepressible, that I did not, could not, become the passive prom queen in demand by the loudest high school boys. But a cocoon can be a silky coffin without metamorphosis. For a long time, I let those boys keep me from believing I could be desirable to men. I was too opinionated, I imagined, too unabashedly competitive, and not about to risk rejection by pursuing members of the opposite sex. Such an attitude deadens one's senses; a woman can't swim in the sea-blue eyes of the man seated across from her on the subway if she can't let herself fantasize about jumping into the water. Gradually, in my twenty-sixth year, I began to realize that I wasn't in high school anymore, that grown-up men could and did appreciate me. Consequently, I began to appreciate them, too. Ironically, my old nemeses, schoolboys, were heralds for the change.

One day about two years ago I drove to work next to a line of boys that started near my apartment and stretched to the lake about two miles east. They seemed to be on some kind of annual trek to the beach. Each wore, or carried, or tied around his head a bright orange shirt printed with the

name of a local high school. They were like a string of bright
Christmas lights. Narrow-chested, toothpick-limbed boys of
thirteen or fourteen; big-muscled older ones who jogged instead of walked, shoulders set, arms pumping stiffly; a sandy-
haired fat boy walking alone; a powerful-looking black boy,
almost a man, also alone. Jostling, joking, bellowing, wres-
tling. This endless line of boys took my breath away, brought
tears to my eyes. The feel of boys, the joy, the potential, the
hope, the bravado. Helen Keller, whose available senses were
legendarily well developed, smelled men's essence in the same
way that I saw it that day: "In the odor of young men, there
is something elemental, as of fire, storm, and salt sea. It pul-
sates with buoyancy and desire. It suggests all things strong
and beautiful and joyous and gives me a sense of happiness."
Until that afternoon in the car, I would not have understood
what Keller meant. I'd always felt left out of some secret club
when women friends commented, "I don't know what it is, I
just like men." That line of boys marched into my heart and
gave me a rushing love of men for the first time in my life
that I could remember.

Where does this leave me as far as my empty black book?
My lover, Mike, is thrilled that I've only had sex with four
men. By his standards, I'm a veritable virgin, and no matter
how much men protest otherwise, they all want to be the only
one. Mike tells me I should be proud. "It shows you respect
yourself," he says. My usual response to this is to roll my
eyes, and sometimes we both start laughing. Respecting yourself sounds so dull. Still, now that I'm approaching thirty, my
lack-of-lovers' lament has become more wistful than a call for
action. I used to worry that I needed more experience so that
I'd be good in bed, but I don't anymore. As Mike says, someone who has a lot of friends isn't necessarily a better friend
than someone with only a few; the same goes for lovers. I
continue to get startled reactions from friends (even my *younger*
sister) when somehow the conversation turns to counting con-

quests, and I reveal my low score. "Only four? You seem like. . . . I mean that's great. It shows you really care about the men you sleep with."

I do feel that I've missed out on something, though. One woman told me that I should feel pleased with my record, considering that AIDS had begun to silently make its way through the population during the time when I would have been sampling a variety of men. On an intellectual level, I understand what she means, but somehow it sounds like a consolation prize. What rankles me is that I may never experience one of those wildly passionate, sheerly physical one-night stands I've heard women describe. They talk about the sparks that flew the moment their eyes met, how they knew they would end up in bed, how they gave themselves over to an attraction that was purely physical. In the end, I believe that glorious, soul-caressing sex has the best chance of happening when you know your partner well and care about him deeply, but if just once I'd taken a lifeguard to bed simply because of the soft blond down on the back of his neck. . . .

Hallmark Holiday

JANICE SOMERVILLE

On our first Valentine's Day together, David and I had just begun to turn our platonic friendship into something more. I was ambivalent about him and the holiday, so I was not too disappointed when the day passed with little notice. I might

234   REINVENTING LOVE

have sent him a card, but although Hallmark seems to carry a line encompassing the full range of relationship situations, I never found one that quite captured my feelings: "You are a real good friend and I liked sleeping with you the other night, but I doubt we have a future."

If he had sent flowers or suggested dinner, I probably would have considered him conventional, unimaginative, and overly interested in me. I imagined us packed into a restaurant, waiters rushing us through the Valentine's Day special, while all around couples gazed into each other's eyes and otherwise fulfilled their annual romantic obligations.

"It's just a Hallmark holiday," David said. "Romance should be spontaneous and inspired, like that night we went down to Hyde Park. It was just a damp, dreary Tuesday night, but we walked for hours. I showed you my favorite buildings and where I had my first job, and you showed me your favorite bookstore. I'll always remember it."

I agreed and thought maybe we might have a future after all.

I certainly didn't want someone handing me a bunch of flowers or a card because I expected it. That would be boring and meaningless, I thought. Besides, the whole idea of Valentine's Day left me cold. I knew it had become a more egalitarian holiday, but it still conjured up uncomfortable images of a long-suffering woman, waiting passively at home for a box of something, anything, that proves she is worthy of being loved.

On our second Valentine's Day, David and I had just broken up after several intense months, and I went to a singles party in Washington, D.C., with my friend Todd. Neither of us had ever gone to such an officially designated event, but this one promised to be entertaining. It was held by an attractive, witty, and highly paid lobbyist, who decreed that every invitee must bring a platonic friend of the opposite sex. We arrived in a festive frame of mind, expecting to meet like-

minded souls—that is, tongue-in-cheek but on-the-make. I envisioned meeting the city's most eligible heavy-hitters and
being ardently pursued by three or four.

At the door was our first indication that this was not to
be. We were greeted by a man dressed entirely in red and
wearing a nametag that said, "Hello, my name is Bob." And
below that he had written, *"Thirtysomething* and skydiving."

"Hi, I'm Bob," he said. "Have a nametag. Write down
two things that you like to talk about."

About twenty people, all in their forties and dressed for
the hunt—the men in suits and ties and the women in high
heels and tight, short, expensive dresses—chatted in the living
room, circling each other and a small table of red food. Red
peppers, red cake, red M & M's, strawberries, and tomatoes
were decorously arranged on a red tablecloth.

I saw my forty-five-year-old self in fifteen years, endlessly
circling tables of theme-party food, consumed and drained by
my single-minded pursuit of male companionship. I left early,
overwhelmed with a hollow feeling, having consumed far too
much red punch in order to convince myself that I would
never come to such an end.

On our third Valentine's Day, David planned to take his
mother out for dinner at an expensive French restaurant. I
decided that was the incentive I needed to bail out. I had
concluded that his winsome devotion to spontaneity reflected
a distaste for planning—but here was solid evidence that he
could, in fact, plan an evening when he wanted to. Immediately, I booked a flight to Los Angeles to visit an enticing man
who had been imploring me to visit.

On Valentine's Day, Chicago was hit by the worst blizzard
in years, and my flight was canceled. I spent most of the
evening trying to get home from the airport. When I finally
stepped off the "el" train into knee-deep snow, wearing a
spring jacket, no hat, and no gloves, I choked back a sob.

None of my friends can come to my rescue, I thought, because they are all home making passionate love in front of fireplaces.

I called David, and he raced over. His dinner had been canceled because of the storm. We walked through the empty streets, the heavy snowfall muffling all sound, until we found an open restaurant. A handful of other people had discovered it, too, and they greeted us like heroes. They beamed at us, and we all shared the secret pleasure of enjoying the snow while the rest of the city stayed home.

On the walk home, full and content, we dodged snowballs thrown by strangers waiting in ambush, and lobbed them back from the safety of snowbanks. Back in his apartment, David opened a bottle of red wine he'd been saving and we toasted each other. He even wished me a happy Valentine's Day. But the evening only whetted my appetite for a true Valentine's Day. It had been memorable, but it had been accidental.

By our fourth Valentine's Day, David and I were happily living together. I still thought too much importance was attached to the holiday, but with my history, I decided I wanted, just once, to celebrate in some small way with a man I wasn't trying to avoid.

I considered planning the evening myself, but decided it would be a disappointment unless he was a willing participant. Not being one to sit back and wait and hope, I decided to take a direct approach. "So, what am I getting for Valentine's Day?" I asked at least once a day for two weeks. "Ha, ha," I always added, so that he would know I was only joking, and that since I was being such a good sport he had better at least get me a heart-shaped box of chocolates.

He winced. "You're not serious, are you? Valentine's Day? How can something that's so contrived be romantic? Can't we be romantic in our own way? We don't need Valentine's Day."

But I had done my homework. "Actually, Sweetest Day is a Hallmark holiday, invented by the same people who make

the cards. Valentine's Day, on the other hand, is a true holiday, which has its roots in an ancient Roman fertility festival
called Lupercalia, and in St. Valentine, who lived in the A.D.
two hundreds and was imprisoned for not worshiping the
Roman gods. The children loved him so much they tossed
messages to him through the bars of his window.

"You like to celebrate Christmas, don't you?" I asked.

He groaned, shaking his head.

I didn't think he would let me down, but he is also a man
of principle. A few days before the fourteenth, he told me he
had a surprise for me. I was thrilled—I love wrapped packages
so much that I don't really care what's inside—but I wondered
if maybe this was a way of appeasing me without having to
plan something. He told me to dress up and that he would
pick me up from work.

When I came down from my office, he was waiting for
me, wearing a red tie and holding a single red rose. The
rest were waiting for me at home, he said. "Pick a door," he
instructed, setting up three numbered paper doors. I chose
Door Number 3, dinner at a French bistro and an erotic movie
at a local repertory cinema. Door Number 1 was dinner at a
different restaurant and drinks at a bar where our favorite jazz
pianist was playing.

Door Number 2 was cheese dogs and TV reruns with
Anne and John, whose company I frequently and futilely tried
to avoid. He told me he had made reservations at the French
restaurant, but that we could go anywhere I wanted. I stayed
with my first choice.

At the restaurant, where they served a special Valentine's
Day menu, we held hands across the table. I caressed his
thigh with my foot, and he wrote a dirty limerick on the
menu. I barely noticed anyone else there. The movie was
deliciously sensual, and when we finally arrived home, tired
and content, we fell asleep in our clothes.

Flirtation

JANICE ROSENBERG

Tim sees the pie I baked for dessert. Cherry, his favorite and I know it. He stands behind me with his hands on my shoulders and says, "You baked a pie. I love you."

"I love you, too," I answer without turning to look at him.

I try for a flat tone of voice, sincere with just the right amount of sarcasm. It's the tone a mother might use—I might use—with one of her teenage sons, a voice that tells the truth without embarrassing anyone.

Tim has been married to Kathy for more than twenty years. I have been married to Michael just one year less. We've been friends as couples all these years and friends as pairs of men and women, too. But the male-female part of our friendship has always been decidedly unbalanced. While Michael and Kathy get along just fine, sharing an interest in music and the usual family-related conversations, Tim and I have been friends from the beginning.

There we were, Tim and I, married at twenty-one or -two, devoted to our mates, but attracted to each other as well. Not that I would have traded him for Michael. I wasn't in love with Tim. But I flirted with him endlessly, and to my delight, he flirted back. When we got together as couples or in groups of friends, I sought him out. I never spoke to him about anything emotional or personal. The times I tried his response was cool, dismissive. Feelings were strictly off limits. He never told me any of his. The one honest part of our flirtation was our true admiration for each other's sense of humor. What we liked to do was crack jokes. Both of us saw ourselves as wits. We had an unspoken rivalry over who could make the funniest ad-libbed remarks. Being funny—silly—had always been my best way of getting attention. With Tim, my jokes had double meanings. So did his. One howler fed another in a kind of hands-off tickling match that left us gasping with laughter. If I was hardly subtle or original, neither was he. His efforts swung wildly between mean teasing and suggestions that we find a motel room. The teasing hurt, but I put up with it and the sexual innuendos, I think, because it was both flattering and fun.

Why did I flirt? Why do most people flirt? For attention, to exercise their sexuality, to prove themselves appealing. Back then I would have said, defensively, that I flirted because I enjoyed it and I could tell that Tim enjoyed it, too. What I didn't recognize at the time was that I flirted because I needed to know that men—a man—other than my husband found me attractive. (Tim was a likely subject. He was equally in need of approval.) I flirted because I suffered from a shortage of male-female experience, having gone exclusively with Michael since I was eighteen. (Tim's romantic history was much the same.) I flirted because I didn't believe that men would accept my serious side and because I lacked the self-confidence to take that chance. (Again Tim filled the bill. His clear lack of respect for women's opinions encouraged my approach.) And, of course, I flirted because it felt sexy.

Although Tim and Kathy moved away from Chicago, we saw them often enough to keep our flirtation alive. Flirting and the anticipation of our get-togethers made for terrific highs and unhappy lows. When our jokes and meaningful looks connected I felt good, approved of. When a get-together passed without some unspecified level of flirtation achieved I went home dissatisfied and grumpy.

Years passed, as they always do in stories like this one. After a Sunday afternoon when we had been particularly overt and both our spouses were clearly upset, Michael told me that the way I acted around Tim had to end. He said he knew it was harmless, but he pointed out how unhappy it made him and Kathy. And he said he didn't want to be friends with them if I was going to continue doing it. He held Tim equally responsible, but he said he knew I could change things if I wanted to. He wasn't confrontational or angry, but he had obviously been thinking about it for a long time and was very definite.

His demand embarrassed me. Were we so obvious? And I was annoyed. Why was he making such a big deal out of this harmless thing? I wanted to change. I didn't want to change. Why should I give up something I found so enjoyable? Something that made me feel so good? Was there anything that I could substitute for it, that would compensate me for the loss? Well, my husband's happiness and my best friend's happiness were two things. But why couldn't they just grow up and accept the flirtation between Tim and me? We'd refined our earlier sixth-grade style to what I thought of as sophisticated banter. It was just a game. Were they too uptight to understand that?

One part of me was angry and resentful, but another part was willing to admit the danger of our game. Or at least to admit that other people—our spouses, to be exact—might not be totally off base in perceiving it as dangerous. Moving along in this mental process, I conceded to myself that this danger was a major ingredient of the fun. What we all meant by danger was the game's undeniable underlying sexuality. And, if Tim and I acknowledged our sexual attraction and considered its logical conclusion, wasn't our flirtation just one long drawn-out mutual seduction?

But this was only one way of looking at it, I argued to myself. Our flirtation could continue unconsummated. Couldn't it? Wasn't it the lack of consummation that created the tension? At the same time, it was the tension, I knew, that stirred up our spouses' objections. There I was, back where I had begun.

To make a long story short, I gave it up. What happened came as something of a surprise. All logic aside, I realized that the game had tired me out. I'd had to be "on" all the time, always ready with a witty comeback, always conscious of Tim's reaction to me. I had to look good, be charming, dress carefully, and seek out time alone with him. By noon on Sunday of a weekend visit this could get pretty old. Maybe this was a rationalization, but I don't think so. If I changed my ways, what I lost by pleasing Michael and Kathy might be somewhat balanced by what I gained in terms of relaxation.

Probably because I'm the kind of person who sees things as either black or white, I went cold turkey on flirtation. The next time we got together I spent most of my time with Kathy. If I made a joke I made it for everyone. I carefully avoided what I had once looked forward to—time alone with Tim.

It wasn't easy. Mentally I stamped my foot and asked why I couldn't have things my way. I forgot what the lows of flirtation had felt like and I missed the old highs, that, yes, dangerous anticipation. What helped me was that the end of flirtation came amid a flurry of other transformations. I was feeling more self-confident. I was feeling less in need of male approval. I was feeling ready for a friendship with a man. Tim was handy. Properly encouraged, he was willing to have a conversation with me. At first I asked questions and he did the talking (just like the dating columnist recommended when I read *Seventeen*). Occasionally we had what I thought of as a tentative exchange of feelings. It was about books or our kids.

It took place in the kitchen doorway or on a walk through the woods with our families. It resembled the kind of talk I had all the time with Michael. If my husband respected my opinions and asked to hear my views of complicated situations, maybe other men—specifically Tim—could do that, too.

Substitutions, sublimations, subconscious reshuffling of emotional needs. For years I flirted with my oldest friend's husband—who just happened to be my husband's close friend—and he flirted with me. We each knew what was going on. We each knew that the other knew. We never once discussed the situation or why it changed. If we did, I'd tell him that I am still attracted to him. Call it chemistry. Call it friendship. If we were the same sex we'd be buddies. We *are* buddies, but underneath, no matter what we pledge to our spouses, the old attraction is still there, so fundamental that we don't need to demonstrate it at all.

In reality, we haven't given up flirtation. We've merely sent it underground, refined it to something subtler. A raised eyebrow, a conversation about baseball, five minutes on the front porch talking while the others get ready to go out to dinner, any of these is enough to reestablish our connection. It's built on years of interaction, remembered incidents, shared jokes, those old days of intense flirtation.

There's something special about our relationship. I think Michael and Kathy recognize this. I think they allow us a certain latitude to be more than just parts of a foursome as our parents were back in the fifties when the men sat together in the front seat and the women sat in back. They trust us now, and that feels good. Our weekends together are warm and cozy and intimate.

Young Men's Bodies

LAURA GREEN

My first year as a college professor taught me more than I
taught my students, since nothing clarifies the mind more than
having to explain the rules you think and work by. That first
season, I didn't just learn to explain the anatomy of a newspaper story. By the time commencement rolled around, I learned
that the quiet rewards of academia were not what I had imagined at all.

They were far more troubling.

I began teaching when I was in my early forties, after
thirteen years on a newspaper and a brief stint as a magazine
editor. Compared to those jobs, teaching was easy, said one
former professor who promised me I could spend my afternoons playing tennis and my evenings doing consulting.
Though my backhand is nonexistent and no one wanted to
pay for my opinions, I did look forward to having more time
to write, flexible hours so that I could see my children, and
a five-minute commute. I didn't foresee the difficulty of mas-
tering a new trade or the stress of concocting entertaining
lectures. I assumed my evenings would be spent with my
writing, not my students', but I spent hours at the dining
room table moving papers back and forth between fat folders
marked "Graded" and "To Be Graded." Most of all, I never
anticipated the distracting young men.

My students, upperclassmen in their early twenties, were as fresh as the morning and as beautiful. Watching those young men stretch their legs out beneath their desks or saunter through the halls was a visual feast that sometimes prompted the most nostalgic, sensual longings in my middle-aged heart.

On hot days, these barely formed men came to my sweltering, un-air-conditioned classrooms half naked in tank tops and cutoffs, their clavicles and shoulders and long, ropelike quadriceps casually visible. In contrast to the young women, who seemed conscious of the way they looked, or would have liked to look, in their summer clothes, the men sprawled offhandedly, arrogantly, about the classroom, slouched down, legs sticking out from under the table, as if they owned the place.

Despite this, they were sweet as colts in a pasture. Their eyes were clear. With their still new skin and barely grown bodies, they sometimes looked the way my own children looked when they were scrubbed and ready for bed. Sometimes the skin over their wrists and palms was almost transparent, with the pink marbling of the flesh that you see in young children. Where the deltoid muscles rose from their collarbones, their necks were as fresh as babies' and as delicate. Their faces were unlined, perfect planes from lower lid to jawbone, smooth as a sheet of flowing water. Untouched by adult sorrow, or so I liked to think. They were so young, filled with promise and time. How could they sense the combination of sensual longing and maternal protectiveness they evoked?

Sometimes I looked across a classroom and felt giddy with their promise. Row after row, face after face, body after body, they sat there, an orchard of young men. I was like the defector in *Moscow on the Hudson*, who is so overwhelmed and astonished by the abundance of choice in a Manhattan supermarket that he faints.

Not that I did anything as dramatic. Not that I said anything inappropriate or put my hand on a young shoulder or made any other intimidating or suggestive gesture. Unlike the Russian defector, I said nothing, took no irrevocable steps. Besides, most of the time, I was too busy teaching to think about it.

Most of the time.

Even though I had long ago learned the difference between thought and act, I was ashamed when I did let my thoughts run on. These students were so vulnerable and so unaware of their vulnerability. As smart as they were, they couldn't imagine they could be vulnerable to abuse or less than equals in a sexual encounter. That may be the futility in a university's sexual harassment code. It doesn't prevent abuse, it only punishes the transgressor after the damage has been done.

I wondered what I would have done if I had been thirty and single instead of in my forties and married.

Still, sometimes, when one of those young men sat opposite my desk, I wanted to reach out and touch him the way I used to touch my husband's wrists in admiration of his perfect body. Occasionally when I was talking to a student after a class, I felt a strong and disquieting urge to put a hand on the inside of his forearm. This unnerved me and I would cut short the conversation and return to my office. It is a wonder I never stopped lecturing and stood openmouthed at the front of the classroom, staring at them the way I used to watch my children as they slept. I wanted to lean over and kiss them the way you kiss a child—for the pleasure of touching something so fresh and soft.

That first year, I watched a much younger teacher who seemed to do what I could never let myself do: desire a student for himself, not out of some mix of nostalgia and aesthetic lust. It was his individuality and his character she seemed to want, not the envelope of his youth. Or so it looked to me as they walked, laughing, along the paths that wound through the campus.

My secret lusts were embarrassing. I was seedy, I thought.

But, oh God, those arms. Those legs. Those flat bellies. If my feelings were common, I'll never know. The women on my faculty were ambitious and discreet. Their eyes were on the prize, not on the students. They were hardly likely to discuss such matters. And even though I had spent most of my working life with men, I was damned if I would ask any of the male faculty if they ever lusted after their women students. I was certain they did and I suspected they lived comfortably with their thoughts and didn't wonder why on earth they had thought them.

I had no desire to be the female equivalent of the poaching professor. At the university, sexual harassment had become a serious matter, and with reason. Hadn't women students come to me, outraged and embarrassed because a teacher was asking them for dates and flirting with them in class? Hadn't I listened and gotten angry, too? Did I want to be in the same league as that guy?

In my own way, I crafted a solution for our times: I fantasized and felt guilty about it. My well-muscled superego made sure I confined my daydreaming to visions of hands touching unidentified forearms or necks or navels or hollows in collarbones. Had I fixed a fantasy on a specific student, I would have been in territory every bit as disturbing as the ground you cover in a recurrent nightmare. It is a dream you don't want. You are ashamed of it. You will it never to recur. But when your guard is down or when you have a perverse need for it, it returns.

Beyond the compelling professional reasons lay the personal ones. I had no interest in betraying my husband. When I began teaching, I had been married for fifteen years and had finally realized that I loved my husband and that I had loved him all along and that he was right most of the time about the things that bound us together. I saw what he had given up for me as clearly as I remembered what I had given up to be with him. I had settled all the scores, often badly, and instead of wanting to hurt him, I now wanted not to.

Besides—and this always yanked my yearnings back to reality—younger men and women represent a great leap backwards. The corollary of a fresh, unmarked body is a mind equally unetched by life. As Gertrude Stein said of Oakland, California, there's no there there. Nineteen-year-old men have nineteen-year-old thoughts, free of perspective and unencumbered by wisdom. I couldn't imagine what I would want to talk to them about other than the material we were covering in the course. What could we possibly have discussed?

I kept thinking about a reporter I knew, who used to tell a suspiciously autobiographical story about a "friend" of his in his fifties who had a lover in her twenties. The problem with her, the reporter said his friend said, was that they had nothing to talk about. Out of bed, she bored him. He finally decided to see her on Sunday afternoons when there was a good football game scheduled. When they finished making love, she turned on the television and watched the game while he took a peaceful nap.

That said, I also believe most older women are less likely to chase after young men because they are embarrassed about their bodies. Who wants to be compared to an eighteen-year-old woman sleek as a seal? Moral scruples notwithstanding, who wants to be compared to women young enough to be our daughters? No matter how I try to convince myself that stretch marks are a badge of honor for giving birth, no matter how I argue that each gray hair was hard-won, no matter how I try to believe that my face is developing character alongside the crow's-feet, I'd rather look like eighteen and think like forty-nine.

This aging does not bother my husband, at least not enough to mention, and certainly not as much as, for example, my habit of picking fights at midnight. To tell the truth, I think we find each other's softness a bit comforting. Or rather, his potbelly gives me permission to ignore a little pot of my own. But I would not have felt that way about his fifty-year-old body when I was in college.

When I was nineteen, and in a particularly lost frame of mind after my father's recent and unexpected death, I had a lover who was twice my age. He was a professor at a commuter college and not particularly well known in his field. Divorced, disappointed, and dismayed, he looked to his students for sexual comfort. He was a bearlike, ponderous man with a barrel chest, a deep voice, and a cigarette cough. He liked bourbon, which, for some reason, seemed more degenerate to me than liking undergrads. Age had not made him a better lover, just an older one. I compared him to the young man I had just stopped seeing. The boy I had loved was as lithe as a cat, and eager, and not yet afraid of life or jaded by it. Sometimes after we made love, he danced for me. My older lover lit another cigarette and groused about his work.

He embarrassed me. I was barely out of high school and didn't know how quickly time passes or how much it means once it is gone. I couldn't understand his fear of dwindling choices, the pain of his missed opportunities or the numbness of thwarted optimism. With the arrogance of a long future, I concluded he was pathetic. And while I remember those beautiful young students with visceral yearning, that fear of feeling my professor's naked need and knowing how much it would embarrass a young lover forever kept me from anything more than dazed wonder.

The Gender Gap: A Fable

LAURIE ABRAHAM

"When I get married, I'm going to move to Aspen and build a log house with huge windows facing the mountains. No curtains," he said to her.

That sounded good, she thought. He was the one who hung curtains on his windows, anyway, sewn by his mother. He had nagged her for months about buying blinds for her apartment. "People . . . [He meant men] . . . can see right in here," he would say as he walked naked from the bedroom to the bathroom. But his double standard about nudity wasn't what was bothering her. It had been one year and twenty-six days since they had heard the orchestra play, since he had unzipped her jeans in the neat woods that edged the lawn where they had picnicked to the accompaniment of Mozart. Night upon night they had spent together since. Day upon day.

Yet he had said, "When *I* get married." Not that she planned on getting married anytime soon. She had never mentioned the word, though she wondered privately how his religious mother would react to her Jim Beam-swilling aunts. Yet it sounded as if he had ruled her out already. Or at most, she had about the same lifetime partner potential as the other 1.5 million women in Chicago. What would have been a better way for him to talk about conjugal bliss in Aspen? she wondered. The most obvious alternative: He could have said when *we* get married. Part of her would have been warmed by that sentiment, but it would have forced her to ask too many questions for which she was not ready. "Does this mean you want to marry me?" would have popped out of her mouth before she could stop it. She did not want to know yet.

He could have said, "When I get married, maybe to you, maybe to another woman. . . ." That sounded more insulting than what he had said. Maybe he never should have mentioned the concept of marriage at all.

She knew if her ruminations about this subject were read aloud she would sound like a desperate man-chaser. That was the problem. "When *I* get married" statements stung her, as they did most every woman she knew. But how could she tell him she did not appreciate being left out of his wedding without his assuming she wanted one? Later that day, though, she could no longer hold her tongue. She told him how hurt she was.

"Oh, I didn't mean anything by it. It's just an expression. I love you, but who knows what will happen between us?"

"What if I had said the same thing to you?"

"It wouldn't bother me unless you had said, 'When I get married it's going to be to a man completely different from you.' "

He looked straight at her with wide-open eyes when he said that. He was serious, sincere, even. It would take a drastic statement like "I'm never going to marry anyone like you"—an accusation more than a statement, the kind of thing you hurl when you are breaking up—before a "When *I* get married" would ruffle him. Incredible.

A couple of weeks later she asked him what he thought

women did not understand about men. "That we're insecure about things," he answered.

"Like what?"

"You know how you told me you joked around with your last boyfriend about the size of his penis. I know you were just kidding him, but it's hard to believe you were shocked that he was offended. Women don't understand how sensitive men are about those things."

"But he knew I was satisfied with him and our sex life. I don't see how that's in the same league as 'When *I* get married.' "

"You're right," he said. "Joking about the size of a man's penis is much worse."

Saying No

JANICE SOMERVILLE

"I'll take you to heaven and back," he told me.

That's not a line I would ordinarily fall for, but he said it in that slightly ironic yet sincere way that can only be delivered with a British accent. And I was still new enough to New York that the deserted, dimly lit nighttime street looked like a set from an old movie.

Daniel repeated that promise several times as we walked from the club where we had been dancing on the Upper West Side. Each time he said it, he looked deeply into my eyes and kissed me, holding me tight. And each time, as we pressed a little closer and swayed a little more, I could feel my will-power drifting further away.

We had spent the afternoon with friends and the evening dancing. Not just gyrating our hips and snapping our fingers, but dipping and twirling in the center of a crowd of clapping people. The last time anybody had applauded my dancing was at the O. E. Dunkel Junior High gymnasium, where I impressed two girlfriends while performing "the Bump" with another. With Daniel, however, I was fluid and confident. My body moved rhythmically with his, matching his expert steps with instincts I had never suspected I possessed.

I vaguely remember talking to him before we danced. I listened to him just long enough to hear a few words (something about Margaret Thatcher and a book he had read), allowing me to check off intelligence. He may well have been asking for a book of matches, but in the event I couldn't help myself and slept with him, I wanted to be able to say that I had liked him for his mind as well as his body and his accent.

As we walked back to my friend's apartment, he gently whispered in my ear how beautiful it would be, using the kind of softly persuasive words that look so ridiculous on paper but sound so irresistible under the moon near Central Park. When we reached our destination, we sat down on the front steps, but quickly rolled over onto the grass. I recalled that my friend, not wanting to disturb her roommate, had brought a blanket into the park and made love one hot summer night.

But a voice from my inner depths was persistent that evening, drowning out my "Life is too short—what is this, 1950?" arguments. I wasn't certain why my puritanical side had the poor taste to assert itself at this particular moment, but I knew I couldn't ignore it. Oh, I could sleep with him anyway, but it would be like having a loudly disdainful third person in the room. Frustrated, I leaped up and mumbled good-night as I ran up the steps to my friend's apartment. I threw myself on the floor next to her bed. My body throbbed. "I'm having some regrets," I told my friend.

"Because you slept with him?" she asked.

"Because I didn't."

Why did I have to choose this night to say no? I asked myself. Why not the night I spent with the guy who had the dollar bills framed on his wall? (Fresh from the mint, the uncut bills were a gift from his mother.) Why not the night with the guy whose favorite and only joke (as I belatedly learned) was: "There's an oyster on your nose!. No, it's not! No, it's not."

I had said no before, of course, and hadn't slept with enough men to shock anyone but my parents. But when the right man came along, I was not one to wait. It didn't particularly matter how long I had known him; sometimes I preferred it that way. And I had never clung to my mistakes, as some people do, punishing themselves or hoping they will learn from them. There are always risks when you follow the unknown, I believed.

Yet shortly before I met Daniel, I had begun to feel that the blunders—the kinds of evenings that make far better stories than memories—were starting to pile up. Separately, they didn't bother me, but they were disconcerting when considered en masse.

The year was 1987, and AIDS was a specter that haunted every casual flirtation. I didn't believe I was really at risk—after all, I told myself, I chose wisely and didn't sleep with too many men—but I thought I should at least become more cautious. I knew it was shallow to feel cheated but I grew up in the seventies, constantly hearing how great sex is and how you should have it often and with as many different people as possible so you don't confuse it with love. And now I was being told I could only have sex in a long-term relationship, which I didn't have and wasn't even sure I wanted.

It was bad enough in the early eighties, before anyone had

ever heard of AIDS, when the media started ringing the death knell for free love and running covers on the new morality. I was still a virgin, and I panicked and threw out my intentions to wait for love. (I was also tired of worrying every time I boarded an airplane that I would crash and die a virgin.)

I had never intended to wait for my wedding night. I just wanted the first time to be with someone I loved who loved me. I wanted it to be romantic and dramatic and worth writing about someday. As it happened, he was gentle and kind, with curly blond hair and a Southern smile, but that's all I remember.

That night, however, gave me a jolting sense of freedom— I could say yes. I was free to enjoy no-holds-barred sex simply for the thrill of it. It was light and exciting and uncomplicated, and it made me feel strong. I could enjoy sex without demands, without pressures, without expectations.

I still believed, though, that sex would be even better with someone I loved. That was the ideal my parents had taught and showed me. They had their arguments, but managed to keep their friendship, love, and sex life alive through thirty-five years of marriage. They had recently moved to a house with a fireplace in the bedroom and a large Jacuzzi, and it seemed every time I called they were either just getting in or getting out of it. That was what I wanted someday, but in the meantime I wanted to enjoy myself as much as possible, albeit while exercising more restraint and more caution than I had.

I was still grappling with these thoughts when I met Daniel in New York. I was so distressed the next morning by my burst of willpower that I wondered if abstinence was worth the sacrifice. A few months went by and then I met Tom, a rugby player, who was cheerful and kind and had the broadest shoulders I had ever held. He surprised me by driving me in his rusty '75 Skylark to his parents' home in Lake Forest, an enormous mansion on the lake. I liked him for that—not for his wealth, but that he hid it so well. He had also once been a masseur, and when he laid me down on an antique bed that he told me had once belonged to a French courtesan, I saw no reason to say no.

Not too long after that, I discovered I had human papillomavirus. I couldn't even be certain Tom had given it to me, because the virus can lie dormant for years. "You should have your boyfriend tested," the doctor said tactfully.

"Is that the only way it's spread?" I asked, hoping he would lay the blame on towels at the health club.

He nodded. "You should also know it has been linked to cervical cancer."

I took a long shower that evening and wondered how I would tell the man I had just started dating. We had not gone to bed yet. "Oh, and by the way, I have a sexually transmitted disease."

I said the words again to myself and scrubbed harder.

Years later I look at a picture of Daniel and me sitting in the sun in Central Park, and although a small thrill still surges through me, he looks very ordinary. I wonder what I missed, and wonder also if he truly would have been the best lover I would ever have, as he promised. And I wonder if he had AIDS.

Pornography

JANICE ROSENBERG

Supposedly, women aren't aroused by pictures of naked men. I keep two copies of *Playgirl* in a locked drawer. Every once in a while, I take them out just to test myself.

I wouldn't want you to think that I bought them for that purpose. Like the men who claim to buy *Playboy* for the great writing, I had my reasons. I bought the first one because I was writing an article for the magazine. (The editor who assigned it retired somewhere in the middle and all I got was a kill fee.) I bought the second issue to read a piece of fiction published by an acquaintance.

The fiction, like the rest of the magazine, focused on sex. If pornography, as the dictionary says, is material that depicts erotic behavior and is intended to cause sexual excitement, I'd say *Playgirl* qualifies. How else would you define pictures and descriptions of men with semierect penises lounging on beaches, or kneeling, muscles flexed, on unmade beds?

When I acquired the first magazine, I flipped past those pages. In an effort to discover whether there was a style formula that my own article should follow, I read "Are You Ready for a New Relationship?" and "Love Language." The articles were reasonably intelligent and not titillating. As for the photos, my attitude was scornful. I didn't need to look at photographs of naked men. Beneath my scorn, though, I was nervous. What if I did need to look at them? Considering all those surveys, maybe I was abnormal. But even if that were true, I reasoned, who would know?

Nobody. I decided there was nothing wrong with satisfying my curiosity. I took a closer look. I considered this research. Did looking at naked men turn me on? Well, yes.

So after my article was rejected, after I read that piece of fiction, I kept the magazines around. Under lock and key, of course. They aren't the kind of reading material you want fanned out on the coffee table when your parents come for dinner. I didn't want my sons to know I had them, either. Let them get their own pornography, I thought. Let them hide those photos of seductive naked women. Let them think their mother would be shocked.

What about *moving* pictures? Are women not supposed to be turned on by them, either? In that case I was in more trouble. When the movie *I Am Curious—Yellow* came to a local theater in the early seventies, my husband and I and another married couple went to see it. Reviews told us that the movie showed couples having sex. I wanted to see it for myself, although I pretended to be interested in the film only as art. And I assume that the others were pretending, too. What we all wanted to see was naked people screwing.

Twenty years later, I remember a misty black-and-white film with subtitles, people speaking inanities in Swedish, the shadowy view into a bedroom where a man and woman could be presumed to be having sex. I don't remember really seeing anything. Or at least not the one thing I'd come to see. I left the theater disappointed, as if I'd bought a ticket for a roller coaster and found the ride tame. Today, *Yellow* is probably classified as "soft" porn, showing foreplay and then, during the act itself, focusing the cameras above the waist or shielding the actors under sheets.

When *Deep Throat* arrived at the theaters, we didn't bother to go. People we knew who saw it joked about the stupid plot and the theaters filled with furtive men in raincoats. (No one ever talks about furtive women in raincoats. Are those surveys right, or are women simply more discreet?) Our friends acted as if those men were sick or evil. I prefer to think of them as more in touch with their animal hungers. In those pre-VCR days what was a discriminating person to do for video entertainment? I soon found out.

I viewed my first true porno movie a couple of years later at that primal setting, the drive-in theater. My husband had convinced me to go, saying we'd have fun. His eyebrows wiggled suggestively. I pretended to be appalled by the idea, but in fact wanted to be convinced. I knew what he had in mind and the idea appealed to me, although I did worry about what the people in the next car would think.

I need not have worried. With our car hooked to the speaker like a deep-sea diver sucking oxygen, we experienced true anonymity. As did everyone else. We were there for just one reason, to be turned on. We focused on the plot, postponing the inevitable, detaching mind from body to savor the anticipation.

Like all the porno movies I've seen since then, the plot served as thin glue between hot and heavy sexual encounters. Scene one: A man is having sex with the adorably lusty maid. His wife discovers them. She is very angry and, it turns out, very uptight about sex, a problem that the generous maid remedies in the next scene. In another scene a collection of uniformly glum friends has gathered at the house for a weekend. In no time at all, the maid has cheered up every one of them. When we left the drive-in we were cheered up, too.

Not long after that, friends of ours acquired a VCR. After a dinner out, they invited us and some other couples to their house to view what they laughingly referred to as a "porno flick." Everyone treated the idea with a kind of offhand disdain, as if porno movies were jokes produced for—you remember them—those furtive men in raincoats. They were like people going slumming, too cultured to admit that they actually enjoyed soap operas or *Wheel of Fortune*, too cool to be turned on by anything as unsubtle as a porno movie.

Knowing how we had taken advantage of our seclusion at the drive-in, my husband and I declined our friends' invitation. They probably thought we were prudes. But the truth was, we couldn't figure out why they would want to watch a porno movie as a group in someone's family room. Unless. . . . No, these weren't the kind of people to participate in orgies. At the time, the VCR was a novelty. I imagined them in the family room, children safely sequestered elsewhere, making nervous jokes about the on-screen happenings, the couples leaving one by one to seek privacy.

Because—is there anyone who won't admit it?—watching people have orgasms (whether fake or real) in porno movies makes you want to have one, too. They are turn-ons just like the photos of naked men and women in those glossy magazines.

When we bought a VCR, my husband and I checked out porno movies on a fairly regular basis. The movies are neatly divided into genres, and, by reading the labels, it was pretty easy to tell what we were getting. We established certain criteria. Neither of us was interested in movies featuring homosexuality, sadomasochism, or child actors. I limited our viewing to movies that weren't degrading to women. (Of course, I had no way of knowing how the actresses themselves were treated, but that's a topic for a different kind of essay.) And we agreed that if a movie turned out to be distasteful to either of us, we would shut it off.

Asking for the movies at the video store embarrassed me. I helped my husband choose, but stayed out of sight while he handled the monetary transactions. I didn't think I was the only middle-class, college-educated woman who watched porno movies, but my truest feelings about them were strictly approach-avoidance. I would have preferred them to arrive at my house in a traditional brown paper wrapper. I wanted to watch them, but I didn't want anyone else to know I did. Sometimes I didn't even want to know about it myself. Yet watching them helped me get in touch with my own sexuality, no pun intended. Over time I learned to accept my voyeuristic side and my attraction to purely physical sex.

Gradually the novelty of watching other people screw wore off. Now we rent a porno movie only once or twice a year. Our all-time favorite is that prototype, *Debbie Does Dallas*. There's something oddly quaint about voluptuous porno stars posing as teenage cheerleaders trying to raise money so that their captain, Debbie, can go to Dallas for a cheerleading contest. The girls find jobs washing cars and selling sporting goods. Each ends up having sex with her employer. In the imaginary world of porno movies—where everyone relishes sex and there are no diseases, date rapes, or pregnancies to fear—it's all good clean American fun.

Of course, my parents wouldn't think so. And, although occasionally I enjoy porno movies, I wouldn't want to make a habit of watching them. Their stimulus is artificial and lacking romance. It leads to egocentric sex. Instead of exciting each other, you and your partner allow the on-screen happenings to excite you individually. For me, the satisfaction of that buildup involves only the most basic release of sexual tension. Although I always turn to my husband in the final moments, I wouldn't call what we engage in at that point making love.

Another thing. Even in the privacy of your bedroom, you're not alone. It's you and your partner and whatever people are on-screen panting and moaning in never-ending ecstasy. Nothing looks sillier than a porno movie once you've gone over the hump. The bodies lose all sensuality and become faceless participants in frantic coupling. You grab the remote control and zap it off. You never know if Debbie gets to Dallas.

The Crush

MAGDA KRANCE

I had a crush on this really cute guy for a year. That's the kind of thing you say in high school, where I was a long time ago, not in married adulthood, where I am now. But there I was, in the throes of a completely adolescent crush (albeit with the perspective of age and experience). It wasn't the first. I have been giddy and silly with longing over guys other than my husband more than a few times over the course of our long marriage (he's had his crushes, too). It was innocent stuff; existing primarily in my imagination, it posed little real threat to my marriage, and gave me great pleasure.

R. was tall, dark-haired, muscular but not overbuilt. His features were perfectly chiseled, animated by twinkling dark eyes. His appeal wasn't exclusively physical, though; that wears thin in a hurry. He also exuded charm and ease and grace. He was generous with compliments. He seemed utterly comfortable with himself and everyone around him. He never showed a trace of moodiness or impatience. He sang professionally. He worked at a homeless shelter. He read for the blind. He was usually broke, but he didn't whine about it— rather, he boasted of the great deals he'd gotten at thrift shops. He could be a mite pretentious, but so can we all.

All this and impossibly handsome, too—almost pretty, but not at all girlish. Well, maybe around the mouth, a little, with those cherry-red lips, that fast and easy smile. But definitely not effeminate. Still, I thought when I first met him a year ago, he might be gay—a dancer, musician, all that stereotypical stuff, and living with a male roommate.

Eventually, in casual getting-to-know-you conversations, there were enough passing references to past girlfriends to deem him certifiably straight. I could now fantasize about him freely, and even flirt with him occasionally, without fear of feeling or acting unconscionably foolish. There's just something gut-churningly embarrassing about discovering that the object of your desire prefers a category to which you don't and can't belong.

So he began to visit my daydreams occasionally. When we actually met we were always friendly, with pleasantly vibrant undercurrents. We sang together in a choir; during rehearsals, I found myself gazing at him dreamily. Some women, and a very few men, are magnets for the eyes like that—simply beautiful to look at and dream about.

And then, one day, mid-fantasy, it hit me: I was too old. He was barely out of college, and I was inexorably approaching forty. By definition I was a matron—married and a mother and no longer anywhere near young. I started to fret: He wasn't flirting with me, he was humoring me, patronizing me even. He was just looking for a ride to rehearsals so he wouldn't have to take the "el" train.

A flush of sadness and oldness and embarrassment threatened to eclipse the delicious heat of pining for him. My romantic fantasies were being muddied by my wanting to apologize for my breasts, which have always been so beautiful and which I'd just noticed had begun to sag a bit, and for the subtle sponginess of my belly since I became a mother, never mind the bags under my eyes. Would he notice, even in my dreams? In my fantasies, I couldn't get past the likelihood of his disappointment, and possibly scorn. I felt that vivid little shock of recognition, the realization that my self-image and the woman in the mirror don't quite match. My ideal self is some pounds thinner and tighter, especially around the thighs, combined with whoever I was in the not-too-distant past, before the gray hairs got to a number beyond counting, before the invasion of the little droops and sags and puffs that come with age. Funny thing; my self-image makeover dwells almost exclusively on things physical, and thus superficial. In all other respects I like myself pretty much as I am.

Still, I see myself as who I want to be and who I have enjoyed being, versus who I am. I think of myself as well toned and athletic, even though the truth is that I scarcely ever have time to run or ride a bike or go to the health club anymore. I don't look bad; I look pretty good, in fact, but I also look my age. As that number increases, the realization has begun to sting.

Getting to know R. and lusting after him focused my mind on these matters more than I cared to admit. As physically perfect as he is, how could he possibly be interested in me, even if only in my imagination? Ironically, there was in our choir a young woman who vividly reminded me of myself a dozen years ago. She and I had similar eyes, and she sported the waist-length dark-brown hair I used to wear. She was also friendly with R. For a while, my thoughts took on a different, more mature turn: They are unmarried and young and beautiful. They belong together. Butt out.

But not for long. At the first rehearsal after several months hiatus, R. greeted me with a long embrace, a friendly (and not too short) kiss on the lips, and the flattering appraisal that I felt good and lean in his arms—that I'd lost weight, which in fact I had. I nearly swooned at the attention. We solicitously asked each other what we'd been up to in the intervening months. And later, when another friend gave us rides home, R. again initiated a long embrace and warm kiss that didn't feel merely fraternal. "See you again at the next rehearsal, if not sooner," he purred.

My fantasies were off and running again at full midlife speed, overtaking my sensible fretfulness. My husband was leaving town for two weeks to shoot the annual swimsuit issue for a national magazine. In doing so, he was the object of much envy and many raised eyebrows, and surely I would be justified in fantasizing about misbehaving a little. In my spouse's absence, R. and I might volunteer to usher a concert. Maybe we'd sit in the back and hold hands. Maybe we'd go out for drinks. Maybe we'd kiss.

In my dreams. The truth was, I had a terrible cold the whole time my husband was gone. R. was the lead in a local production. Even if we'd had time to get together, I couldn't risk getting him sick during the opera's run—even in my dreams.

At a subsequent rehearsal, we shared a tangerine during break, along with some lingering looks. We went off to wash our sticky hands, and found ourselves in a private washroom, alone. It was a perfect moment for a stolen thrilling kiss, a shared secret to replay repeatedly with half-closed eyes and parted lips like a lovestruck teenager, and to grin at each other about for weeks afterward. In my dreams.

What does all this giddy silliness mean, and where does it come from? I'm clearly old enough to know better. I am contentedly married, and no, contented doesn't mean dead. My husband and I are wonderful companions and domestic partners. As parents, we're often too tired for sex, but it's terrific when we get around to it. We are secure and stable and happy. I am not looking to replace him with anyone.

Ah, but sometimes the soul—mine, anyway—needs to long, to crave, to pine. I can't pine for someone I already have, so I find some bright new object of desire. Not that I'm ever looking, but sometimes, it just happens; I encounter someone, in this case, R., who took my breath away. Fantasizing about him was like taking a tiny cost-free vacation from the routines and responsibilities of my grown-up life. It was a regression to adolescence, to vulnerability, to the possibility of romantic adventure.

Unlike a lot of adolescent and single-adult fantasies, however, my current daydreams were zipless and futureless. I have no interest in imagining any kind of settled life with R.; I already have that. The point was to dream of passion and abandon.

Those dreams were deep-sixed when R. told me his "Michigan honey" was coming to visit. Young and cute, no doubt. I sank back into my matronly mode again, even feeling prudish in a reverse-double-standard way, as if it were inappropriate for me to have prurient thoughts about him because of his distant romantic attachment.

But not for long. Good fantasies die hard. We continued to flirt in a friendly manner. R. fanned the flames with casual references to recent and current flings, and with his easy physicality. We massaged each other's backs during rehearsal breaks and before performances. Then one night I noticed a few gray strands in his thick dark hair—a surprise, considering his youth—and he complimented me on my gray hairs. We smugly agreed that the idea of hair coloring was unappealing, not to mention too expensive, and that neither of us is so insecure as to need to hide our gray.

Then I asked him a question I thought I knew the answer to: "How old *are* you?"

"Thirty-one," he piped. "But I act sixteen. And I got carded last week."

My heart fluttered with delighted surprise. With only five years between us, I suddenly stopped feeling too old.

Lingerie Limbo

JANICE SOMERVILLE

My college roommate Tracy was packing to spend the night at her boyfriend's house. Opening her dresser drawer to select underwear for the evening, she slowly surveyed the rows of lacy, creamy, satiny panties and bras that lay inside. An ivory sachet separated each tidy stack.

Light as tiny, silky parachutes, the lingerie seemed to float into her hands. First the virginal whites, then the courtesan reds and blacks. Some were entirely sheer, and some were mere strips of silk. A faintly lush fragrance wafted into the air.

Tracy was having sex, and wildly, too. I opened my drawer after she left. Crumpled next to my T-shirts lay a wad of beige Carter's briefs, which I had worn since childhood. They're practical, comfortable, and they wash well, I told myself. I had seen Tracy hand-wash each of her pairs of panties, then hang them on a little line she strung up in the bathroom. I didn't have the time for such extravagances, I reminded myself. I had also seen the price tag on some of her underwear, and I knew she had to select each item separately. Carter's came in convenient, inexpensive six-packs.

Why was I envious? After all, I sometimes envied Tracy's long, shiny, red-polished nails, but I had never been able to hold my nails still enough to keep them from smudging. There were many things I was supposed to do to make myself more attractive, but I stubbornly kept to the basics—mascara, blush, and a blow-dry. The rest were unnecessary and often painful, like high heels and plucked eyebrows. Sure, Tracy's underwear looked sexy, but how long could you wear that stuff? What's the difference if they're just going to come off, I asked myself. Just because some guy liked them didn't mean I was going to walk around with my butt up in the air, trying to get comfortable. He would just have to accept me as I am.

Not that anyone had ever asked me to wear something sexier.

I knew I was supposed to want to wear them for myself. But I did not particularly want to feel the caressing touch of silk on my body, reminding me that I was horny and alone, which was depressing enough. It might also lure me into bed with the wrong man.

I was comfortable, and none of the men I subsequently dated suggested I change. Until I met David. He wasn't critical, just baffled that I found beige sexy. "They're comfortable!" I protested. "And besides, they're flesh-toned. Anyway, I like them."

"Well, I'd like to see you in something sexy."

I felt a vague tug of defensiveness over my Carter's—my last link with my tomboy past, when life was simple and lived only for myself. But I also envied Tracy's lingerie drawer. And I did want to excite David.

On a rainy Saturday afternoon, between a workout at my health club and a stop at Ace hardware, I slipped into the door of the Lingerie Factory. I felt like an impostor among the women who rummaged so casually through the piles of panties. I spotted a pair of peach silky ones that cost as much as an entire package of Carter's. I bought them quickly and ducked out the door.

When I tell this story to friends who have grown up on satin-panty Christmas presents, they look at me strangely and

suspiciously. But I was not uneasy about the lingerie or about
sex. I was uneasy because everyone else seemed to belong
there, and I didn't—and I wasn't sure I wanted to. What else
might I find myself doing? Using rollers? Giving up beer? It
was the same feeling I had on the two occasions when I had
presented my stubby, ragged nails at a nail salon, or when I
once found myself seated on a stool, having eyeshadow applied
at a department-store makeup counter.

That feeling quickly passed, however, as David's response
made me a regular at the lingerie store. Since then, I've gradually amassed a large collection, some of which is not even very
comfortable. I have the usual assortment of Victoria's Secret
pairs, a Christian Dior matching set, lacy bras, and so forth.
I also have several pairs of Jockeys for Women. I buy the
French bikinis in several different colors. But they're cotton
and they come in sets of three.

Perhaps it seems painfully obvious that I was reluctant to
become a woman, but I don't equate femininity or maturity or
even sensuality with lingerie. A *New York Times* article recently
pointed out that Calvin Klein, when he created cotton underwear for women in the early 1980s, "liberated women from
fussy lace and polyester silk undergarments."

But the truth is, I now like fussy lace and polyester silk,
whatever that is. And I like cotton. Fortunately, I live in a
time when underwear is no longer a moral or a political statement, and I can be like the strong women in the Jockey ads,
or a sex object for the man I love—and he can be a sex object,
too, in the silkiest, skimpiest pair of black bikinis I can find.

At least in my dreams.

Lingerie Anxiety

CARROLL STONER

I didn't quite know what to do about the beautiful red silk underwear my husband gave me for Christmas. Intellectually, I accept that wearing elegant, expensive lingerie should make you feel elegant and expensive. Obvious, right? The *Cosmo* girl might compare it to keeping a bottle of champagne in the refrigerator to remind her to celebrate and make her feel worldly and dramatic. Lingerie should give you similar feelings, only sexual: It should make you feel seductive, desirable, beautiful. Even if it just sits in your drawer with sachet tucked into its folds, its presence should sit reassuringly in the back of your mind.

The reality is something different. Let me back up and explain that I've bought myself about a ton of beautiful sleepwear and undergarments over the past decades. I remember as if it were yesterday buying that first pair of bikini underpants in the grown-up lingerie department of the best store in town when I was about fifteen. Wearing that red underwear made me feel daring, sexy, as if I had a secret, long before anyone but girlfriends saw what I wore under my clothes. As for sleepwear, I've worn long, sexy black nightgowns. I've owned a white lace and tricot nightgown and robe set that was virginal when I was not. I've bought vivid print bras and underpants, pastels and darks, tailored and a little frilly. Once, in the weeks before my son's birth, when I couldn't work or do much of anything, I sewed a nightgown and robe out of beautiful fabric. The enforced leisure made me slightly crazed, so I poured my energy into an incredibly elaborate ensemble for the hospital and afterwards. Under ordinary circumstances I am a fast, sloppy seamstress, more interested in effect than details. But that outfit lasted for years because it was sewn with total devotion. Every seam was perfect. Both the gown and the robe looked as beautiful inside out as on the right side. Because I sew, I know that good workmanship and fine fabric are tied to price. Well-made lingerie is expensive and it lasts. Show me cheap lingerie and I'll show you something that will end its life in the ragbag, and not too long after its purchase. To work for me, lingerie must be durable enough for the washing machine—which is one of the reasons I got myself in hot water with the red silk stuff.

The source of my guilt was three pieces of beautiful cherry-red underwear lavishly trimmed in taupe-colored lace. Heavy, lustrous satin. Silk satin. Incredibly elegant, the deep red color was somewhere between rambunctious and glamorous. I thought I was uncomfortable about them because the care label said, "Hand-wash and press with a cool iron while still damp." Would I do that? Could I burden my once-a-week cleaning lady with such an intimate task, therefore letting the living room go undusted? Everything in life is a trade-off, but this one seemed more painful than most. As much as I wanted beautiful lingerie, could I rationalize wearing a camisole, half-slip, and underpants that cost more than my first car? I was not working at the time, which surely influenced my dilemma. Some of us are not cut out to be pampered ladies of leisure.

Complicating my problem is the fact that I hate the idea of returning gifts. For the most part, I give gifts to people I care about. I take it seriously, attempting to buy things that convey a message, that they will use for years, and that they wouldn't buy themselves. Lavish silver ice buckets, a ward-

robe of vases for a lifetime of flowers, an antique something—
my choices are carefully thought through. I expect the recipient to accept my gift with grace. My husband gives gifts with
the same forethought. His first wife returned every gift he
ever gave her, which doesn't surprise anyone who knows her.
She preferred giving him a shopping list of items in specific
shops, which amazed me with its unembarrassed crudeness.
When he told me this, I remember thinking I'd never do such
a thing.

Could I break my own rule? Could I return that beautiful
lingerie?

I did it. And got a hefty credit. I think I bought sports-
wear, but am not sure, which says a lot about taking back
gifts that have been carefully chosen for you. He told me,
more sadly than I care to remember, that he saw me in those
things. He loved the red, he said, although he had debated
between it and black. It was a vision I was not able to share.

An earlier attack of lingerie anxiety was caused by my first
husband, with whom I had profound differences of opinion
on everything in the world, from whom we should eat dinner
with to what we should eat for dinner, not to mention whom
to vote for and why. But nothing tells more about our differences than the turquoise nightgown and peignoir.

The nightgown was simply cut and hung from spaghetti
straps in long, full layers of semisheer fabric that swirled when
I walked. The matching robe had flowing, wide-cut sleeves,
and both the neckline and sleeves were trimmed in marabou
dyed a brilliant, matching blue-green. I was stunned by this
gift and could hardly wear it, feeling as I did like a clean-cut
twenty-three-year-old masquerading as a gangster's wife. The
ensemble was glamorous and beautiful. But what would I have
worn with it? My fuzzy slippers? No, I'd need velvet mules
with a little heel. I'd have to fix my hair before I put the
gown on, or maybe slip into a platinum wig. This wasn't
lingerie. This was a lifestyle. I kept the outfit for years and

finally gave it to a baby-sitter who thought it was the most beautiful thing she'd ever seen. I was glad to be rid of it.

I also remember struggling with what to wear for a romantic tryst in the Caribbean. It would have been too brazen to go there with nothing in my bag to wear at night. I was meeting a man I cared about (though I had no intention of marrying him), a man who had made me feel desirable and loved after a marriage when I'd felt neither. He would be in Florida on business and had planned a long weekend for us at an island resort. I shopped. And shopped. For someone with an extremely limited attention span for shopping, I went all out. Stopping in at least three Fifth Avenue stores, I learned a lot about the merchandising of lingerie.

There were lovely pastel nightgowns with tiny, appliquéd roses, delicate embroidery, and little bows at the neck, which were entirely unsuitable. I wanted him to hand me a glass of champagne, not a lollipop. At the other end of the spectrum, there were black nightgowns with see-through lace bodices that were so . . . blatant. I knew even then that they were for husbands who need a little jolt and like seeing their wives' lace-covered breasts. Fine. But not for me. I bought a short, leopard-print nightshirt, which was not perfect but at least didn't make me feel idiotic when I put it on.

Maybe I have a limited imagination? One of those "I-couldn't-possibly-sleep-in-*that*" women who refuse to recognize that sexy sleepwear is donned to be removed, not to be slept in? Naaaa. I love playing dress-up. I've been a sucker for sequins, and I recently bought a full-circle taffeta skirt that was perfect for the dance floor, no matter that my husband and I never go dancing. I've had clothes fever, that fever accompanied by breathlessness that can befall a normal woman when she sees something so beautiful that her heart stops and her own psyche is replaced by some alien force that takes over and absolutely . . . must . . . have . . . this dress/sportswear/ pair of earrings. I once bought an Escada outfit (gorgeous!) on a credit card while I was in San Francisco at a conference, spending two weeks' salary on an outfit that I thought would change my life. It didn't, of course, as I knew it wouldn't when I regained my sanity, but the event so shocked a colleague that she still mentions it ten years later. No, I can be a fool for fashion.

A friend cuts to the chase. "You're from Minnesota," she says. "You can't possibly buy into the images of men in smoking jackets and women in flashy lingerie. They're foreign to you. Minnesota is plaid wool robes and fuzzy slippers."

I think she's right. Although one part of me wants to sit at a dressing table with a mirrored top and a tray of antique perfume bottles while I brush my long, wavy hair with a sterling-silver-backed brush, the real me has straight, wash-and-wear hair, is in a rush, and sprays from a prepackaged bottle I order once a year from a catalog. I know there are people who can feel natural wearing ascots and velvet jackets. But mostly, I think they live in their own imaginations, since the idea of an American monied and leisured class rings false to me. I believe the first thing a rich person with any sense would buy, after a great house and a few vacations and some fabulous flowers to be delivered weekly, is an interesting job.

Lifestyles for women in incredible lingerie suggest gliding through a perfect house with everything in place. I, on the other hand, stride. I am purposeful. I would snag a three-layered peignoir on a piece of wood as I threw it on the fire, maybe going up in flames in the bargain. I don't languish on a perfect bed. I conduct my late-night life (what little there is of it) from a slightly messy one. My bed is for talking on the telephone. In it I read novels and newspapers, fight over the TV remote control with my husband, eat herring on Ritz crackers and think it's a wonderful substitute for caviar on an English biscuit. I believe anyone in her right mind would prefer a Triscuit over a water biscuit any day of the week.

My trousseau was not full of hand-sewn silk dressing

gowns. Life is not a romance novel. I do not swirl through
the room in a cloud of floating fabric to get myself—or him—
in the mood. I guess, when you come down to it, I don't
think sex is theater, and therefore I don't want to wear a
costume for it.

Fortunately, the same man has known me intimately for
over twenty years, and we have begun to envision each other
through collective eyes. He has great taste, and once he accepted my somewhat practical nature, things began to work
out. I like luxury, but only to a point, as the red satin lingerie
proved. Now, he buys all my sleepwear and lingerie and says
he enjoys it. My favorite is a deep magenta-colored gown that
is cut on the bias, slit up the sides, and fairly low-cut but still
respectable in case I run into my son or daughter while wearing it. It came with a matching jewel-toned, striped satin robe
that has magenta lapels and piping that match the gown. We
went shopping together for this, and I insisted on poly-silk
rather than the real thing. Polyester may not sound elegant,
but it's practical, and today's designers do wonderful things
with the details. That set has been in and out of the washer
and dryer for several years and has many more years of wear
left in it. Although it is far from being worn out, my husband
recently bought me a replacement, an equally beautiful gown
and robe in flowered fabric by the same designer.

I love lingerie, but I think it means more to him than to
me. I like him to do the choosing. It's like sending him to the
grocery store to buy the luxuries I am incapable of putting
into my shopping cart. I used to think it had something to do
with self-esteem and that I should learn to buy my own expensive lingerie. Now, I like it because it says he cares enough
to give me great stuff, and because I'm happy with his image
of my sexuality.

ENDURING LOVE

Sweet Talk

Sweet talk ought to come naturally. For some adults it seems
to, but how did they learn to do it? Even if their parents
talked plenty of sweet talk to them, I doubt that many children returned the favor by calling their mothers darling.
Clearly, if they are to grow up as spontaneous sweet-talkers,
children need someone to practice on.

That's why I think every child should have a dog. Oh, I
suppose a cat would do as well and I have heard my kids
whispering to their hamster, but a dog is what I know best.
Dogs are perfect repositories for sweet talk. A dog isn't offended by silly baby words. He isn't embarrassed in front of
his friends if his name is Sarge and you call him Poopsy. Dogs
like to take long naps and during these naps they give every
appearance of appreciating any affection that happens to come
their way.

I like hearing my seventeen-year-old son call our German
shepherd sweetie. I've never heard my son call anyone else
sweetie. He gets down on the floor nose to nose with the dog
and, patting his broad head, murmurs, "Are you feeling okay
today, little sweetie? I hope you are. You're such a nice
doggie-do. I love you." Then he kisses the dog, calls " 'bye"
to me, and swaggers off to high school.

When we were first going together, my husband, Michael,

wanted me to call him intimate names. He longed for en-
dearing epithets and I couldn't supply them. Oddly enough,
after the first time, I never had any trouble with "I love you."
That's direct and so am I. But standard sweet talk felt saccha-
rine and phony. And he wanted more than a casual "babe"
stuck at random into a sentence. He wanted oodles of sweet
talk, gobs of it, great armloads of what at the time I was
simply too uptight to give. I had no practice in the subject,
no experience. The closest I could come was an occasional
"Mikey," which, looking back, makes me cringe.

If, as a kid, I'd had a dog the whole issue would never
have come up. "Oh, cookie, lambie doodles, little honey," I
could have crooned, remembering how I scratched my dog
behind his ears. "Oh, dolly pie, itty bitty poochie baby," I
could have murmured, recalling how I'd stroked his fur. But
without the benefit of sweet talk experience I was lost.

When I was a kid I wanted a dog the way teenage boys
want cars, the way pilgrims in the desert long for water. My
parents saw a dog as a general nuisance, a mess-maker, a noise-
maker, an addition to their newly built suburban home they
could easily do without. It would chew the rugs and leave
brown pee spots on the grass. Or vice versa. Sure, it might
give a sense of responsibility to my brother and me, but more
likely it would just create endless situations for kid-parent
conflict.

My parents did not know what they were depriving me of
when they refused to buy me a dog. (And, at the time, it
didn't occur to me that a dog would give me anything but its
undivided attention.) More to the point, they did not know
what they were depriving me of when they failed to call me
honey. Nicknames and diminutives were the closest that anyone in my immediate family ever came to sweet talk. My
father called me Jan-Jan. He called my mother Ruthie. An
all-purpose dear (used for his patients when he forgot their

names) occasionally slipped from his lips. My mother never, ever, not even once by accident called me anything but Janice.

I remember only one relative who handled endearments easily. My aunt called me lovey and it was wonderful to hear. For years I connected the word with everything about my aunt that was warm and caring. She called me lovey, so I knew she loved me. It didn't hurt that she was also a great hugger with a super lap for cuddling into and a deep bosom to rest my head against. Even with four children of her own, she had plenty of affection left over for me. In my childhood, lovey belonged to her alone. I never thought it was a word that I could use. At my house it would have sounded as foreign as Greek.

I suppose the lack of sweet talk in my childhood home was directly connected to my parents' uneasiness with any of their emotions. I rarely heard my father cheer at football games. When jokes were told, he never let loose with truly uproarious laughter. And he discouraged it in his children. When we were growing up he was forever telling my brother not to laugh, talk, or complain so loudly. At family get-togethers he still exhorts my brother and me to calm down when we begin to warm up to an argument, even if the subject is as impersonal as who should be the next mayor of Chicago.

My mother is equally reticent. She was surprised and hurt when, as a college student, I told her that I thought she never worried about me. She never worried *out loud*, she said, but she worried plenty. Although I didn't want a Nervous Nellie for a parent, I would have liked to hear a few of her worries. Like sweet talk, worries serve as an indirect but highly audible expression of a parent's love.

My mother did eventually learn to call me dear. Better late than never, I suppose. I noticed it on the telephone one day shortly after her first grandchild arrived. "It was nice talking to you, dear," she said. And a few weeks later, "I'm sorry that happened to you, honey." She sounded stiff, like someone

practicing for amateur theatrics. But I didn't comment. It was
a start.

Over the years, the words have become more natural on
her lips, and she's expanded her sweet-talk vocabulary to include the word "love." As in, "Give my love to Michael and
the boys." I can't help wondering: Does she ever tell anyone
else to give her love to *me*?

Of course, there are people who use sweet talk too cheaply
and freely. To some waitresses every customer at the diner is
honey. To some construction workers every woman who
walks by is sweetheart. These words lose their meanings when
they're used too often or with strangers. But between a parent
and a child the words are like warm touches, quick connections permeated with deeper feelings.

I want to tell my mother, it's not good enough to assume
your child knows you love her. Daily reminders are necessary!

My father is no better with words. I suppose he never will
be. The other day on the telephone I said, "I love you," and
he said, "Thank you." On the other hand, he has always
been a good hugger, a sincere hand-holder, and an enthusiastic
supporter of even my smallest accomplishments. That com-
pensates.

So there I was all those years ago, directly out of a non-
sweet-talking family, dating a boy in dire need of sweet talk.
In his family darling and sweetheart were as common as bread
and butter. His pet name for me when we were eighteen was
French—*mouton*. We didn't discover until much later that it
meant sheep rather than lamb.

I didn't realize I should be calling him something special,
too, until he said, "If you can't call me darling, there's something wrong." He didn't accept my explanation that I simply
wasn't comfortable with words like that. He couldn't believe
that they didn't become part of my spontaneous repertoire
once I loved him.

To please him, I went through the motions, hoping to

learn by doing. I worked the occasional word into a question, as in Have you taken out the garbage, dear? I managed to tack darling onto I love you fairly often. But my best opportunity for practicing sweet talk came after our first son was born. If a dog doesn't do it for you, a baby will. (Or should. With my mother, for some inexplicable reason, it was a grandbaby.) We called our new son Daniel, but not too often. Mostly it was Spaniel, because nothing else rhymed (and I still didn't have that dog). We called him Tweetie Pie because with his skinny neck and round face and wide-open eyes he reminded us of the cartoon canary—and that led us to Sweetie Pie. We called him baby and softened it to bee-bee. (One day we made a list of all his pet names and hung it on our bulletin board. I wish I had saved it.) Our second son started out as Gabriel but on his first day home we called him Gaby-baby and in no time shortened that to Goo-goo. We called him Goo-goo for a long time and still occasionally do, although he's seventeen and doesn't appreciate it.

Or so he would like us to think. But I know how much I like to be called Jan-Jan by my father, and to this day, when my aunt calls me lovey I feel warm all over.

As for my endearment deficit with Michael, instead of continuing to stumble over the standard terms, I did what I had done naturally with the kids. I invented my own. They've varied through years. Lambie-pie, lambie-lou, and boo-boo rank high among the current favorites. Honey-pie and lovey (which I now claim for myself) round out my vocabulary. At less creative moments I resort to a simple sweetie. It sounds good to me.

Mortality

MAGDA KRANCE

I'm getting to an age at which mortality is a real concern—but not mine as much as my husband's.

At thirty-seven, I'm still fool enough to assume that I'll live forever. Steve, however, is an insulin-dependent diabetic approaching forty. His body's graphic declaration of mortality was a horrible jolt more than a decade ago, when his Type I (formerly known as "juvenile") diabetes was diagnosed. We were young then, if not exactly juvenile, but suddenly we both knew what is almost certainly going to be the cause of his death, although not when or exactly how.

Day to day, it's not a major issue, but it is an undeniable presence. "How's your blood sugar? Are you low?" I ask if Steve starts to act at all strangely—if he abruptly becomes very gregarious or expansive or speaks in non sequiturs or becomes glassy-eyed, as if he's had too much to drink. If he's not too far gone, he pricks his finger and puts a drop of blood on a tiny strip of chemically sensitive paper. If his blood sugars are indeed low, he eats or drinks something—usually rather noisily and grossly, though I've learned that this is not the time to nag about drinking directly from the juice jug or wolfing ice cream straight out of the carton. Not that it doesn't annoy the hell out of me when he stokes his furnace with Ben & Jerry's, Godivas, or the last slice of homemade cheesecake—

delicacies meant to be savored, not merely gobbled—instead of some more run-of-the-mill fuel. At other times his blood sugars are high, and he feels and acts sluggish until he injects some extra insulin. Syringes and alcohol swabs are as much a part of his daily self-maintenance routine as a toothbrush.

In general, my husband is in excellent health. He exercises, eats well, and takes his condition seriously. There's no reason not to assume we'll both live indefinitely, at least in theory, and continue to do somewhat meaningful and satisfying work—he as a free-lance photographer (well paid) and I as a writer. Still, there have been some bad scares in recent years, some harsh foreshadowings of his mortality and its possible consequences.

Several times Steve has slept through or worked through the early-warning signs of hypoglycemia—low blood sugar—the condition which, if untreated either with juice, a soft drink, a glucose tablet, or in severe circumstances, an injection of glucagon, can result in unconsciousness, seizures, and death.

The first time it happened, we were in Wisconsin, visiting my mother for the Fourth of July. I woke around 5:30 a.m. with Steve thrashing in bed next to me, his arms flailing, torso rolling, and head snapping. His eyes were darting and glassy. Was he having a nightmare? a seizure? I could barely understand what he was saying. Mostly he just mumbled an echo of whatever I asked him: "Steve! Are you having a nightmare?" "Naaaaghtmaaaaare," he answered, slack-jawed.

I called the local hospital and was told to get either juice or a soft drink into him and to call back if that didn't work. I ran down to the kitchen; uncharacteristically and distressingly, there was no juice in the fridge. Fortunately, there was a can of Coke—pure providence, as none of us drinks the stuff. I grabbed it and ran back upstairs. I poured some into a glass and held Steve's head up. He'd stopped flopping around, but was now too disoriented to drink from a glass. I ran back downstairs, managed to find a bendable drinking straw, and ran back up. "Suck!" I yelled at him, as I propped up the dead weight of his head and shoulders with one hand and held the glass in the other. That reflex remained, at least, and he obediently drew on the straw. Swallowing was another matter; he coughed and sputtered, but managed to get some of the drink down. I'd also brought up a banana and some chocolate, and fed him bits of each as if I were feeding a pet.

And then it hit me: What if this is it? What if he's had brain damage, and this is how he's going to be from now on? What if he never snaps out of it? God, he's only thirty-seven— how long could he live like this? What if I'm pregnant? What are we going to do?

He, meanwhile, was looking at me with alarm and terror in his eyes, but through a sort of cloud. He seemed to realize that something was terribly wrong but could do nothing about it, as if he were floating out to sea on a chunk of ice, beyond my reach. I had seen that look before, the remote and panicky helplessness, in my father's eyes when he was sick with a brain tumor.

I told Steve to move his hands and legs. Weakly, he lifted his right limbs a few inches. His left side, though, was immobile. His eyes widened in horror. I lifted his left hand, but it flopped straight down as soon as I let go. He had no control of that side of his body. I called for an ambulance.

By the time the paramedics found my mother's country hideaway some twenty minutes later, the Coke had kicked in, and Steve had come back from semiconsciousness. He was terribly weak, but he could sit up and even move his left side a little, although not enough to stand or walk. His head felt thick, he said. He talked haltingly, bemusedly, about what had happened in the past hour, which had transpired almost as an out-of-body experience for him. "What if I've had a stroke? What if I can't work again?" he asked with heartbreaking bewilderment.

By the time we reached the hospital Steve was still weak but his mental faculties were pretty much restored, as evidenced by his exasperation with the patronizing patter of the emergency-room physician, who knew less about diabetes than the patient. Still convinced he'd had a stroke, Steve insisted on a CT scan, and got one. The results, fortunately, were negative. Not that the news was all good. Apparently, he had had a seizure, and a temporary bout of unilateral paralysis—an unusual response to extremely low levels of blood sugar.

Steve later asked his regular doctor, who specializes in treating diabetes, if any brian damage might have occurred. Possibly, the doctor replied, but it would be nothing detectable in a CT scan. Instead, he said, it might affect Steve's subtler senses and capacities—his appreciation of beauty, his creative abilities, that sort of thing. It was hardly a reassurance. Also, the doctor said, having this kind of episode made it more likely that more would occur in the future—that Steve's ability to recognize the onset of hypoglycemia and treat it on his own might diminish.

Nevertheless, we eventually lapsed back into normalcy and routine. What else was there to do? It's like looking for lightning—you never know when or where it's going to hit until it's happened. And nothing happened for more than a year. We conceived and had a little boy. Steve was the model father—loving, enthusiastic, involved, responsible.

Then it happened again, when our son was just a few months old and starting to sleep through the night. I woke around four in the morning with Steve groping me in a clumsily sexual fashion. He was humming tunelessly, with mindless cheerfulness. Crossly, I nudged him away and told him to be quiet, but he continued to hum and mumble and grope. But this wasn't dreamy ardor; it was severe hypoglycemia. I turned on the light; he continued to blither and hum, glassy-eyed, semiconscious. This time I was angry more than alarmed. He had checked his blood before bed and had declined to have a snack, and this was the result. It needn't have happened. I wanted to blame him for not managing his health better, even though it wasn't his fault; he is as scrupulous about it as possible.

I slapped him hard on the legs and belly, but he just kept humming insanely. I jammed a straw into a box of juice and made him drink it, so mad that I couldn't look at him. When I did, there again was that blank, needy stare. I fed him a banana and more juice. He continued to babble, then finally fell asleep.

I, of course, couldn't. I was utterly wound up, flushed with anger and adrenaline. What damage had been done this time? What would happen if we were apart and this happened, if he or I was away on business? What if I wasn't there to minister to him? What if he was taking care of our son when this happened?

In the morning Steve woke up well rested, with no memory of the episode. I exploded from the stress and worry and lack of sleep. It wasn't fair to be angry with him, I realized; these episodes are no more volitional than are the seizures of someone with epilepsy. But I couldn't help it. Crying and shouting, I told him that it scares me to death when this happens. It strains my caretaking capacity. The nerve-fraying stress and anxiety linger long after the episode has passed. It terrifies me that he can so easily drop off the edge. What would I do, what would we do, our son and I, without him?

That is no small matter.

In spite of the women's movement and the supposed great strides we've all made professionally and economically, the twenty-second nightmare fantasy flashes through many women's minds as we and our mates age and mortality becomes more than just a distant specter: What would I do if he had a stroke? a heart attack? How would I get the kids through school on my income alone? How would I manage without his love and companionship and support, financial and emotional?

"Whenever my husband is ten minutes late coming home from work, I'm convinced that he's dead," confided a friend who was pregnant with their second child. "I tell myself that I'll move in with my mother, have the baby, and go back to work, and somehow, we'll make it—and then he walks in the door and we have dinner."

Because of Steve's diabetes, though, the twenty-second what-if nightmare is more than a passing frightening fantasy. For me, it's a strong likelihood. I don't dwell on it, but I can't ignore it, either. Because of it, I looked for and found a full-time job, the kind with a regular paycheck and decent benefits, the kind into which I hope I can settle. It's a depressingly grown-up thing to have to do, after years of letting serendipity guide my career and life—a luxury I enjoyed because Steve's income allowed it—but to put it off much longer is to court disaster.

Steve had several more extreme hypoglycemic episodes over the next several months. They were like little fires, perhaps not deadly in themselves, but terrifying in their implications. Each time, for as long as it took to grapple with him, get him to drink some juice, and wait for his blood sugars to rise, he literally became another person—a frightening, irrational stranger in my husband's body.

Particularly terrifying was the episode that overcame him not in his sleep but one evening when he was taking care of the baby while I was out. I came home late to find Steve sitting in the kitchen in a state of incoherent agitation. "Iiiiii'm jusssssst tryiiiing to keeeeeep thissssssss plaaaaaaace togetherrrrrrr!" The words squeezed out of him like something on an altered soundtrack. His arms flailed as he spoke. He looked mad at me for not understanding. Increasingly agitated, he repeated his non sequitur responses and gestures. I walked around him and found our son, then about eight months old, asleep on a jumble of toys on the floor. Furious, I scooped up the baby, laid him in bed, returned to the kitchen, and dished

up some ice cream and a glass of milk, which I ordered Steve
to eat while I stormed off to wash up. How could he be sitting
in the kitchen and not have the presence of mind to feed
himself? How could he neglect himself when I wasn't there
to keep an eye on him, and most important, when he was
taking care of the baby? How could I ever leave them alone
again? It made me wonder if I could afford to be out of the
house, away from him and the baby, even as much as a regular
job would require. How often would I have to call in to make
sure everything was okay?

Then, somehow, it stopped. Or at least it hasn't happened
for some time now. Somehow, Steve regained the ability to
respond to his lowering blood sugars before they dropped too
far—to wake up out of a deep sleep when his heart starts
racing and make his way to the kitchen alone.

Contemplating the continuing reverberations of those severe hypoglycemic episodes has led me to a series of contradic-
tory realizations about the life and lifestyle I've taken for
granted for years. It boils down to this: I resent, at least
slightly, being taken care of, but I also resent the possibility
that I *won't* be taken care of.

In most respects we are a nontraditional couple, or a new-
traditional couple. I cook; he sous-chefs. He does most of the
grocery shopping and laundry. We both take care of our son;
Steve probably changes more diapers. In most respects we
have a true partnership. Financially, however, our circumstances have been very traditional. He is far and away the
primary income-earner, a fact I do not relish but have come,
reluctantly, to accept. I am mildly bothered at not having the
sense of empowerment that comes with a substantial income.
As a feminist and professional who has been committed to
free-lancing for more than a decade, I'm frustrated that I
haven't done better financially. In the past two years, though,
that double sting has been lessened somewhat by having be-

come a mother, and having to accept the challenge of that essential and thrilling (but nonpaying) new role.

On the other hand, the baby's arrival, coinciding with Steve's out-of-the-blue hypoglycemia problems, has sometimes given me a sense, right or wrong, of being the family's ultimate gatekeeper and caretaker. On a day-to-day basis, of course, I know I'm not. Steve is a wonderful provider and partner in the mundane tasks of daily life when he's well, which is most of the time. And he, I know, feels that the burden of the family's well-being rests on *his* shoulders, as he is the one who pays the bulk of the bills and manages the finances.

Still, because of the nature of his condition, because low blood sugars affect his brain and thus his judgment and behavior, I feel as if I always need to keep tabs on his status, to make sure he's really okay, to make sure that all bases are covered. I feel like a supervisor, a manager, a delegator. Steve may shop for the groceries, but I'm responsible for the list, for knowing what's needed. I sometimes feel as if I have to be on call at all times for the baby's cry and for the possible recurrence of my husband's hypoglycemia-induced temporary insanity.

When it comes to caregiving and caregetting, there's a very fine line, and a chasm of ambivalence, between loving attentiveness and resentment, and between loving acceptance and frustration. In normal times, we all need to be needed—to a point. And we all need some amount of care—to a point. When things aren't normal, though, points move and lines blur. Everything changes, more often for worse than for better. The caregiver can easily burn out. It can take considerable effort and patience to do what needs to be done cheerfully when illness or impairment brings down one's partner. And it's no picnic being on the receiving end, either, especially in a society such as ours, with its heavy emphasis on self-reliance.

The caregetter can become distressed and embittered at any loss of autonomy and ability.

But let's face it: Risks are part of the big gamble of love and marriage. Life together *is* a burden and a responsibility—for Steve and me, for anyone. Marriage comes with the pledge to support each other in sickness and in health, for better and for worse, for all its joys and pleasures as well as for its unforeseen complications. Most couples have little need to think about what those words really mean at the time they utter them. Sooner or later, though, we all find ourselves staring down a long, lightless tunnel of mortality with that vow reverberating in the darkness. What we do then, whether we manage to bail out, whether we stand by one another or flee, is the ultimate revelation of who we are, and whether we have truly become adults.

Having contemplated the long-term prospects for our marriage and our family since Steve's first bout of severe hypoglycemia and our son's birth, we have made some accommodations in our lives we might otherwise have put off. I have taken a full-time job, which, fortunately, I quite enjoy, with a financially stable company. For the first time in my working life I have a reasonable salary and benefits—and Steve is covered by my health plan, preexisting condition and all. Taking the job represents no small change of lifestyle after a dozen years of free-lancing, but it also represents a liberation from the resentment I'd felt earlier at the possibility of being left alone, essentially helpless financially, as has been the case for too many wives for too many generations. It would, of course, be crushing to lose Steve, and I pray it won't happen. But I know now that it would not be crippling. I would be able to survive and support our child. Facing mortality before it's a done deed has, I guess, made me an adult.

Equal Partners

CARROLL STONER

When I left my job in a hurt and angry way a few years ago, I wasn't aware of how everything in my life would change, especially my marriage. Looking back, I know the upheaval was related to the fact that power and money have always been underlying themes in my life, and that they had become important in my marriage, especially in my financial contribution to the partnership. The real problem, though, was that I was unwilling to face any of it.

At first, being home was sweet. I got over the psychic exhaustion caused by a corporate takeover and the chaos that followed. For three months I didn't want to do a thing other than create order at home and spend time with my husband and children. Fabric samples, games and movies with my kids, cooking and running all the errands that kept our domestic life operating became my major interests. Then something happened. I'd always believed that home and family were acceptable ways to express yourself, but what I found was that however true that might be for other women, such expression only works for me when it's done in tandem with work. Paid work. My career had become so closely linked to who I am that without it I began to . . . drift is the best way I can describe what happened. I thought I would, for the first time in my life, be able to relax and let myself be taken care of, but for many reasons, that did not work out.

I know I shouldn't have to justify loving success. Men have traditionally measured themselves by their achievements and women by their husband's and children's accomplishments. In the new, improved world we are supposed to create, women would change that by somehow being both highly successful and less materialistic. We are supposed to care more for our families than about our jobs, as if some final "Sophie's Choice" between them might have to be made. I love my family, but my salary and the public role of being a recognized newspaper editor also mattered. Because of family ties, I couldn't move. Practically speaking, redundant newspaper managers at my level look for jobs in other cities. Once before we had moved for my job. Now, my husband had a well-established business of his own and there was no question of uprooting everyone. So there I was.

In retrospect, it seems fairly clear, as it must to marriage counselors who are familiar with the impact financial issues have on relationships, that my earnings had become central to how I feel about myself. It was more than money. Without a job, I wasn't the woman I wanted to be, or the wife my husband expected. We both had gotten used to my income, we spent up to it and, yes, we needed it.

My husband resented my ability to walk away from a job (even one that had become untenable) and, at least on the surface, never look back. He couldn't do that, even if he wanted to. Now, our entire livelihood depended on his income. I couldn't face his anger. It made me feel terribly ashamed of what I perceived as my failure. "It wasn't my fault. I've always taken care of myself, and I still can," I wanted to shout, even though it was no longer entirely true. On the other hand, "Men should be able to support their families," said a small, clear voice from another era that still lived inside me, the same subconscious voice that said it was easier to blame someone else than to examine my own situation.

I hadn't just worked throughout my adult life. I had held a job or owned a business since I was the seven-year-old Christmas-card-sales champ at Our Lady of Victory Elementary School. My parents took me out of the Catholic school system but I kept the business, and from that point on I'd enjoyed financial independence, literally never having to ask anyone for money. I learned to balance my studies and work; later, when I had children, I had liked managing a busy life.

To say my work was important to me is to vastly understate the case. People have always told me I'm a lucky person, as if all the jobs I've loved have happened by chance. The truth is, I've worked hard to find and succeed at those jobs. And I love the entire process of work. But when I found newspapers, I found the perfect career. My love for the fast-paced business became an addiction: The people are smart, the work a series of quick takes that offer instant gratification, the adrenaline rushes delicious.

By the time I was in my forties, I had a lot of responsibility, managed a big group of sharp people, earned a good deal of money, and was proud of it all. Maybe too proud. At some level, I'll always be a small-town girl whose father wasn't successful and whose mother was ambitious. I was happily married and loved being a mother, but the most notable part of me was that complicated drive to achieve. And the downside of the ambition was that I had begun measuring myself in terms of public validation.

To complicate matters, my husband kept telling me how well I was handling things. What he meant was how little I spoke of missing my newspaper life, how little I worried about my future, how little I complained. On some level, this was simple stoicism. The unwillingness to face difficulties goes back to my upbringing; in my family, we were expected to keep a stiff upper lip. I am also a genuine optimist, sometimes to an improvident degree. The combination of optimism and stoicism is not good, and in the same way I'd faced my parents' deaths in my twenties, I now closed off all emotion about the loss of my job and simply did not speak of it.

In the bigger scheme of things, I told myself my little career and the marital problems that developed were not important. There was a great big world out there, a world that contained hunger and war and poverty. All the "self" words that give women so many problems came to mind. I was being selfish, self-centered, self-pitying, self-absorbed. I beat up on myself and absolutely refused to take my emotions seriously, unwilling to face the fact that, however unfair it might be, my career as a newspaperwoman was over. Feelings have lives of their own, I have since discovered, but at the time I told myself I just had to get out of myself and find a new place in the world. What I would not face was how angry I was about my situation. And in the way that such buried emotions always show in one way or another, my husband was bearing the brunt of it.

To make a long story short, by the end of several years without meaningful work, I was seriously adrift. I started a business and sold it. I bought some country cottages, fixed them up, and made a nice return on my investment. I found that I love the bottom line of business, a surprising discovery for a journalist. But none of this brought me either the satisfaction I needed or the weekly corporate income we'd grown used to. And in the meantime, a new pattern began to take hold in my marriage. I was frustrated, powerless, silent, and angry, without ever articulating why. He was feeling the strain of having to pay all the bills.

No matter what amount of money he gave me—willingly, never asking questions about where it went or questioning my financial judgment—just having to take money from my husband killed me. I wanted my own income. I wanted a seriously challenging new career.

While I was nursing my grievances and wounded pride and feeling overwhelmed and depressed and financially dependent all at once, I kept myself on a short purse string. I boasted about how thrifty I was, telling a friend that I could save money in a thousand little ways, including using my husband's discarded razors rather than buying my own. Of course, these money-saving techniques made me feel even more impoverished. Any therapist in the world would have seen how I was punishing myself, but since I wouldn't see a therapist ("Nothing wrong with *me*!"), I missed seeing it myself. I watched food bills (the only thing I could really control) like a hawk and completely eliminated prepared foods in favor of doing it all myself, carrying my enjoyment of cooking to some new, martyred extreme. Doing without was easier than facing my needs. At the same time, I ran all the tiresome family errands that needed to be run, which only added to my feelings of resentment and frustration. What had once been done by paid help, or sandwiched between bigger events, now took up entire days. The kind of work I'd loved was no longer available to me, and unwilling to take the kind of job I could get, I threw myself into solitary writing. My husband, in turn, worked longer and longer hours.

Time spent together dropped to next to nothing. Conversations about anything meaningful all but disappeared. Our sex life sagged. It's hard to make love to someone you'd like to throttle. Even our sacrosanct Wednesday-night date, the time we had for years scheduled to spend together, was totally forgotten. I blamed him for not making plans and he blamed me for something unspoken—probably for no longer being any fun to be around. We spent evenings apart. He watched television. I worked or read or slept.

The image of these years that will linger in my mind is of me huddled over my computer, writing, writing, writing, trying to figure out what had gone wrong, hating my life, and using him as a scapegoat for everything. I had married the wrong man, I told myself. If only he made more money, I rationalized, I wouldn't have to think about what had happened to me.

Let me emphasize here that his earnings were never in question. He is a hard-working, successful, self-employed businessman, good at what he does. The sudden drop in income was mine. How did it happen that after all those years of enjoying my earnings and working to increase them, I suddenly expected them not to matter?

We fought. We made up. We fought again. We made up. And then we started fighting without making up. The word "divorce" was mentioned in the heat of several of our arguments. For at least a year things were very bad indeed.

And then, when things couldn't be any worse, a few small things began to change. I remember waking up one morning and looking across the two feet of space that now separated us in our queen-sized bed. I began to think about how happy we'd once been and how well suited we'd once considered ourselves. And I thought, "He's a good guy. You're being too hard on him. And on yourself." As I lay there, propped on my elbow and watching his even breathing, I faced the fact that I had two choices. I could put some time and energy into it, insist he do the same, and keep our marriage going. Or I could end it. The enormity of my choice was right there and it almost took my breath away.

We could not, under any circumstances, get a divorce. It would hurt our children deeply, and our daughter was only eleven. This was a second marriage for both of us and we are too stubborn to admit failure. We'd invested close to twenty years in our marriage, many of them sweet years. We'd loved each other and had been close, loving friends. Couldn't we recapture that? On the other hand, we had stopped liking each other. My friend JoAnne, stuck in a bad marriage for close to twenty-five years before she found the man she recently married, says she thought her marriage was normal until she met us. "I never knew it could be like that," she says. "You were so *nice* to each other." She gave me some advice. "Stop worrying about Bob. Get your own act together. *Get a job!*"

A close friend who is divorced told me repeatedly to work on my marriage. She cautioned me that unless I had a specific reason to break up—and he'd better be rich and good-looking—I should work things out. Then, too, if we broke up, my husband's ex-wife would have the last laugh. No, divorce was out of the question.

As I lay there, he threw the covers off his long, slim legs, woke up, and asked, "Are you okay?" I started to cry and he put his arms around me and I whispered, "Why can't we just be nice to each other again?" And he whispered back, "We can."

So did we live happily ever after? Not quite. I dragged him to a family counselor, which he saw as an admission of failure, but I saw as a sign of hope. It worked. After screaming at each other for several months ("I see a lot of hurt and disappointment here," the therapist said), we realized that articulating our problems and facing them meant we could finally see some solutions. I need a job. He needs a wife he considers his equal. Because of who we are, we constantly struggle for power in our marriage. But without a sense of equality, I had begun to give in too easily and the delicate balance that defines our relationship was upset.

When my book business took hold and checks started rolling in, the healing process began to speed up. My confidence returned. We started to talk about business again, and we began to listen to each other on that and other subjects, as we had in the past.

In the long run, what I learned about our marriage is what I needed to learn about myself: As much as I love my family and home life, the sense of achievement I get from work is essential. I like having money as a way of keeping score. I also like having what it buys. I had to face the fact that I both

crave and resist being taken care of. It upsets some deeply
held belief in myself. It makes me depressed. The reality is
that when I'm not making money, I can't feel strong or independent or satisfied. My ego is dependent on achievement. I
know there are many women like me.

I also know that I don't make a good martyr. I hate running everybody's errands, and when I see women who have
built their lives around all the mindless little tasks it takes to
keep a home and family running, I feel sorry for them, even
when they don't feel sorry for themselves. I love running my
home, but don't find doing so meaningful enough to occupy
a lifetime. Errands fall ridiculously short in terms of the passion I need to aim at something worthwhile. Sure, I know all
about taking classes and finding meaningful community work.
But I've been spoiled by my own success. I want to work on
my own terms.

Since I feel more responsible for our domestic and community life than my husband does, I must earn enough to pay
someone to take care of some parts of it for me or I get trapped
into doing it all. That had been a major bonus of my financial
independence. In the same way that he used to depend on me
to keep our domestic life running smoothly, I had always paid
someone to take care of home chores. In my marriage, equality
means sharing in the financing of our life, as well as sharing
in the emotional caretaking that goes into every relationship
and family. No matter what else happens, without the earnings that guarantee clout in marriage, our partnership can't be
successful.

I have also learned—and this may be the most difficult
thing of all—that when bad things happen they must be faced
and grieved over. Only then can they be left behind. For the
rest of my life I'll have to remind myself of that, since I have
a tendency to bury the bad news and keep smiling. I learned
that even if I have to force it—as I probably will, since my
husband, like most men, does not seem to have the same need

for communication that I do—we must talk to each other and discuss our feelings.

I always knew, but had forgotten, that I must have a marriage of equals.

Insomnia

MAGDA KRANCE

We lie here, back to back. You sleep, your breathing deep and regular, a comfort and an annoyance both. I want to be swimming in sleep, too. But awake, I'd rather have the close rhythm of your breaths than have the bed to myself.

I arch a little so we press flesh, butt to butt. That nuzzling touch does not rouse you. Nor does it lull me back to sleep. My brisk heartbeat accompanies the relentless march of mundane thoughts parading through my brain: Write the Christmas cards. Clean my office. Send out these clips and query letters. Cook the beets for the baby. Freeze the chicken breasts.

I try to will this herd of mental lemmings off a cliff. They will not go. I turn, burrow, nuzzle you now with a heel, later with a knee. Your sleep is not contagious on contact.

This begins in deep darkness. The street is silent. I have nursed and rocked the baby and laid him down again. Perhaps he sucked the sleep out of me. I drink the still water in my bedside glass, and settle back down. It doesn't work. The light outside rises, traffic gathers, and sleep still refuses to overcome me.

So I listen to you breathe, deep and slow, envying your slumber but savoring your closeness, your reassuring breathing. I try to take your pace, and think about how this, far more than passion, is the essence of our union—breathing together, sleeping (or not sleeping) together close and contented. If I can't have sleep, I'll settle for this profound and fundamental comfort.

Just the Two of Us

JANICE ROSENBERG

People ask me all the time what it's like now that it's just the two of us. My younger son went away to college this fall. My older son started his third year away. Of course they come back for vacations, but our old, reliable, everyday family group is no more. It lingered in a nostalgic form when the older one was away and the younger one still home. When I told people how sad I expected to be when he left, how I'd be all alone, my husband, Michael, always asked, "What about me? I'll be here."

I confined my worries to how I would get along without my sons, never considering the issue of how I would get along *with* my husband. Two-ness wasn't something we had a lot of experience with. We were alone together for only three years before our first son was born, and in those years Michael was a medical student and then a resident who spent more time at the hospital than at home. When he *was* home he often fell into a sleepy trance over dinner.

We never had the romantic extended honeymoon that a friend describes as something she and her husband are looking forward to resuming when *their* kids are both away. She describes having spent entire days in bed, and, although she's too discreet to say so, I imagine them making love—as well as watching old movies, ordering pizza, reading tidbits of *The*

New York Times to one another, cuddling together in their warm cozy bed on what I assume were winter Sundays.

We don't have that to return to because we never were exactly what you'd call a couple of adults getting to know each other, either before or after marriage. Our courtship and early years were more a growing up together, which is why being just the two of us means that, sometimes, now that we've returned to those free days, we return to being kids.

On a recent Monday afternoon, for instance, we went to Chicago's Museum of Science and Industry to see the latest Omnimax wraparound movie, *Antarctica.* We arrived with time to spare, so we went to our favorite place in the museum, the gift shop. We rarely buy anything beyond a postcard, but we both like to look at the toys and books and remember which ones we wanted but never got when we were kids. This time Michael admired a clear plastic replica of a human body and told me how that toy had inspired his medical career.

Our interest in souvenir gift shops, the unself-conscious way we hold hands, our sentimental affection for psychedelic rock songs are positive results of growing up together. But growing up together led inevitably to separation. We became like children pulling away from parents, working to be ourselves.

Let me explain.

When our marriage began, we went grocery shopping on Sunday mornings, invited single friends as guests for dinner, and never would have considered seeing a movie with someone else. When it came to activities, Michael was the leader. When he wanted me to share more of his interests—biographies of politicians, beginner's tennis, tropical fish—I went along. (Years passed before I noticed that this was a one-way street. I never thought of asking him to join me in one of my interests—sewing, cooking, painting, or ceramics. That wasn't the way it worked. My interests were meant only to keep me busy when he wasn't around.) An inveterate hobby taker-upper, Michael worried that we didn't have enough interests in common. Because I worried that he might be right, I let myself be dragged into activities that I cared nothing about. I felt guilty about saying no, because I knew he thought that "no" meant I didn't love him. Or anyhow, I thought that was what he thought. We rarely told each other the truth about our feelings. Thus, when he started spending time at an indoor archery range, I went along. When he learned to fly, I took more than the lessons necessary to make me a competent emergency backup, even though I found it terrifying.

One of the reasons I went along, however grudgingly, was that I couldn't stand for him to have fun with someone else. Sometimes my acquiescence worked out okay; he suggested skiing and we both enjoyed it immensely. But he wasn't supposed to enjoy it without me. Once, when I was six months pregnant, he went to Wisconsin with some medical school buddies for a day of skiing. There was no way I could go, and so I didn't want him to go, either. And when he said he was going anyhow, I did my best to make him feel bad about leaving me. I sulked until he left, then lay down on the couch and read all day, books being the barrier that I've used all my life to stave off loneliness.

Loneliness in one day? Yes. I could sink to the depths in a matter of minutes. My loneliness had nothing to do with reality. It had nothing to do with entertaining myself. I really did like reading. And there were friends I could have called, plenty of old movies on TV, sewing projects. There were museums, for God's sake, and movie theaters and musical performances a bus ride from our apartment. None of that mattered. I was so insecure that the shortest separation hit me with the force of total abandonment. It was a visceral response of lostness, uncontrollable, tear-inducing. I had married Michael believing he would be with me forever—and constantly.

And so it went. Michael remained the leader. I followed,

coming to resent his power over me, learning only very slowly that my own neediness gave him the power. It took much longer to see that his power trip revealed a depth of neediness in him as great as mine.

I could get analytical here, talk about our parents' marriages, their ways of loving us, examine in detail why teenage rebellion came over me after thirteen years of marriage. I could lay out the messy details, tell you what my rebellion did to Michael, how he fought back, how I fought back. It wouldn't be pretty.

Instead, let's just say that eventually, the shoe changed feet. I grew stronger and began to pull away from him. Then he was the one who wanted every second of my time. When I took an evening writing course, he insisted on arriving at precisely ten o'clock to pick me up. If I turned down his offer he called me ungrateful, so I complied, allowing him a surface remnant of his old power. Inwardly, I seethed with the itchy indignation of a child whose parent has her on a too-short leash. Busy with my sudden, separate growing up, I failed to note the possibility that he, too, feared abandonment, perhaps had feared it all along.

When things grew tense beyond our abilities to cope, the therapist we saw said that we were merged, a condition that turns sour when one partner begins to feel claustrophobic. Which I had. Gradually, we focused on things we would each do alone or with a friend, separated those from the ones we truly enjoyed doing together. I had my writing friends. He had his flying companions. We enjoyed art. We liked to ski. And most important, we really did love each other. All our interests didn't have to be the same.

As the time drew close for our second son to go to college, I worried about a relapse into dependency. I remembered my past reactions to being left behind, and, for a week or so after we dropped him off at school, I had all the old symptoms. I felt abandoned, not just by him, but in general. I cried at odd times and needed lots of hugs and reassurance. I hid out in books. My emotions mirrored those I'd had in childhood and in the early years of our marriage. Understanding that they were triggered by my son's leaving, but were hardly reasonable emotions for a grown-up woman, I had the strength to fight them.

Fortunately, Michael knew how to respond. He tolerated my teariness and my need to be with him. When he went out to the record store, a place I have no interest in, I went along. Every morning for a week or so, I woke up lonely. But I knew better than to glom on to Michael permanently. Those old ways weren't healthy for either of us. So I comforted myself with other things—new books, shopping expeditions, essay writing, work, and female friends.

Michael didn't really understand my feelings—"Children grow up, they go away to college. It means you've done a good job as parents and you should be happy"—but he willingly supported me through them anyhow. I am the one most obviously susceptible to dependency, but Michael, who, like most men, has few confidants, is vulnerable, too. Now that it's just the two of us, the idea of having him dependent on me for all his human contact is almost as frightening as the idea of my becoming, once again, dependent on him.

When I think about long-married (happy) couples, two competing thoughts cross my mind. First, how lovely to imagine the infinite connections and depth of understanding they must have with one another, and, second, how frightening to have one person so important to you. One half of every couple must certainly die first, and to survive alone, the other must have the strong interior self that dependence doesn't provide. The solution to this paradox is that being deeply important to one another is not the same as being dependent.

Lately, without ever having discussed the subject, each of us is working to allow the other extra space. Each of us has been doing more things separately with friends. Mostly we arrange these plans so that they don't take up the time we like to spend together. Not because we feel guilty about time spent apart, but because we honestly enjoy being together. There's a new casual quality about our relationship, yet we're in touch on a deeper level than ever before. As with trees planted close to each other, our branches spread out on their own, but our roots are firmly wound together. While we might go to the movies with someone else, neither of us would think of taking a vacation without the other.

We have our rituals and routines. We watch the news at ten. We take the dog for walks in the park. We listen to music and read. With a raised eyebrow one of us can remind the other that no one's home and we're free to "play," which is our way of saying let's make love.

No matter how we've spent our weekend days, we share an early-evening cocktail. This tradition comes from Michael's family. I thought it terribly urbane the first time his father offered me a mixed drink at five on a Sunday afternoon. Michael's mother served sprats on Sea Toast. We have potato chips or pretzels, or, for a special treat, mixed nuts or sesame sticks from the candy store on Broadway. Michael always has Scotch on the rocks. Most of the time I drink bourbon and soda. Occasionally I switch to a very dry Spanish sherry or a glass of wine. We each have one drink, sipping and crunching at opposite ends of the living room. We switch from classical music to jazz or folk or Broadway show tunes, put our books aside, and talk.

It's not perfect, being just the two of us. We still argue about whether I'm too bossy or he's too sloppy. If we're angry with each other there's no one to talk to at the dinner table. We both know that, and so our arguments are shorter. We like to have them settled before we sit down. Now that our younger son is away we can talk about subjects that interest only us, without having to consider whether he feels left out.

We can talk about people he doesn't know without explaining who they are. We can tell each other the same old stories without anticipating his sigh of boredom. Best of all, we can talk about our sons. Or simply eat in companionable silence without the pressure to use mealtime for interacting with our kids.

We were partially prepared for this two-of-us routine by independent children. Before they went away to college, they left us on our own a lot. Even when they were younger and needed us to be home with them, Michael always had Monday off. For years we've spent Monday afternoons together, just the two of us, doing everything from simple errands to flying over the countryside looking at autumn trees.

They say when your parents die you lose the wall that separates you from death. I feel something similar about my sons' departures. Their gradual moving away has removed the wall that separated us from middle age; it has opened the vista of being on our own together, made us think more about the concept of forever.

While I don't think either of us feels that our marriage is in danger, there is a precarious sense that with the kids grown it has lost one of its main reasons for existence. We still love each other, but we know that people can easily be tempted from safe harbors by passion or romance or some other less easily defined enticement. A longtime couple has to renew the decision to be together, and, quietly, that's what we're doing. With our children no longer needing to be nurtured, we're nurturing ourselves—and our marriage.

True Love

LAURA GREEN

They were mystified out there when my husband and I got married. I can see why. He is silent. I am voluble. I have to stop myself from finishing everyone's sentences. He likes to watch people talk. I am a serious cook with shelves of cookbooks. He'll eat anything but sweet potatoes or raw meat. He loves explosion movies and war movies and martial-arts movies. I hate them. When I saw *The French Connection*, I cried when the subway conductor was shot because he looked like a family man. My husband says higher mathematics is like poetry, that you can write an equation that will turn a rubber ball inside out. I have no idea what he is talking about. I can fill in most of the countries in Europe on a blank map. He can recognize Italy because it sticks out like a boot. He never looks back. I cannot let go of the past.

For vacations, he wants to rent a houseboat and motor down the Rideau Canal in Ontario. I want to rent a house in Greece. I want to go to East Africa or the Amazon; he's thinking of visiting his sisters out West. I dream. He acts. He'll see the world before I will.

He is a tall, blond, blue-eyed Californian, all legs. His ancestors were whaling ship captains and pioneers, people who crossed the prairies in Conestoga wagons and sailed around the Horn. I am short and dark, all mouth, a Slavic Jew whose grandparents came through Ellis Island. His grandparents knew Pancho Villa. Mine knew the managers of the traveling Yiddish theater.

He is a natural athlete who can watch a ballplayer on TV and imitate his swing because he knows by watching how the moves will feel. I cannot hit a tennis ball across my own court. He is so confident he once lashed himself to a mast to help get a boat back to harbor during a sudden, violent squall. I am a coward who canceled our hot-air-balloon ride so many times that the man finally sent my money back. I can't swim in water over my head without wondering if I will drown. He does somersaults off the diving board and never thinks he will hit his head on the bottom of the pool and break his neck and be in a wheelchair forever. When I tell him that when he is late I wonder if he is dead, he looks at me as if I am crazy. Maybe I am.

That is what they said when Steve and I got married. My friends assumed we were carried away by lust. My sister swears that one Thanksgiving—maybe it was the year we slow-roasted the turkey and didn't eat until almost midnight— she watched while my husband and I, kissing and oblivious, slid gradually from our chairs under the table. I remember no such thing. But I do know that we found each other's differences mysterious and appealing, as if we were puzzle pieces that knew they would fit together.

Yet though we were certain we loved each other, we were acting on instinct. Sliding along on sexual momentum, we confused infatuation, which comes out of nowhere, with friendship and loyalty, which are built brick by brick with more false starts than a cathedral. But when I married him, it was enough to know that when he saw me in a room he felt my presence the way I felt his. We were satisfied with the mystery of one another and had faith that a communion deeper than fascination might follow. What optimists we were!

Despite the undeniable chemistry that drew us together,

we were an unstable combination in a stressful life. The first few years, he was working long days at a hospital and I was running back and forth between my job at a newspaper and the baby-sitter's. When he was home, he was asleep, trying to gather his strength for the next round of thirty-six hour days. When I wasn't at the office, I was raising two children and running a household on the fly.

Exhausted and swamped, we fought like cats in a bag: about housework, about money, about why he got to nap and I didn't, about why he never called his mother and father, about the way we made love, about those silences I had once found so intriguing. When I think of those early years, I remember us in our old apartment in bed. I can feel the wrinkled sheets, see the mess of magazines on the floor, smell the car exhaust from the busy street just outside. The couple in the apartment above us is making love again, rocking their bed against the wall with a low, steady thump. Thump. Thump. Thump. They go on forever, thump, thump, steady as a heartbeat, dull as a metronome, reproaching me for my anger, for wanting my husband to be someone he is not. Unlike them, we are fighting again. I weep and scold while he lies there silent, immobile, suffering, refusing to give an inch.

"Why won't you answer me?" I cry. "Are you afraid to talk to me?"

"What is the point?" he finally says; then he pauses and adds from the bottom of his fatigue, "Just what is it you want me to do?" His voice is so weary that my heart goes out to him. I want to hold him, but I do not. He would only roll away from me.

After a day or two of silence, one of us tiptoes up to the other to say, "I'm sorry. I don't want to fight like this. I love you." I put my arms around him or he puts his around me and we hang onto each other like survivors. Survivors in a marriage.

Given that I had married Steve for his differences, how

did they come to irritate me so? Why did he always have to mispronounce "facade" so that it came out "fasscade?" How could he keep confusing Robert Service and Robert Lowell? Why did he keep asking me to go to Japanese movies? Why couldn't he like what I liked? It seemed to me that my tastes and style were clearly superior to his. Once he was exposed to them, he should have found them irresistible. But he didn't. He stayed the same absent-minded, competent, independent soul he had always been. He didn't care about style; he cared about skill. I had married a man who could build a back porch in an afternoon but got lost driving home from the lumber-yard. My husband was oblivious to style, but I needed its diversionary potential.

His favorite movie demonstrated the differences between us. *Tokyo Story* is as slow-moving and laden with meaning as a tea ceremony. As I recall it, a quiet couple work their farm and raise their children. They don't say much and they don't go anywhere. The high point comes when they are old and sit on a dock all afternoon, motionless, silent, whole. Steve's eyes practically got misty when he talked about it, so moved was he by their wordless communication. I knew this was what he wanted for us and the prospect dismayed me. I wanted fun, energy. I wasn't ready for depth. I yearned for a husband who ate Vietnamese food, liked to talk, and jogged—in short, a husband who was just like me. Poor Steve. I couldn't accept him even though he accepted me. What was worse, I didn't understand why, if he accepted me, he didn't want to be more like me.

Maybe what held us together was Steve's faith that we were the same at heart. That and our fear of divorce. We had both buried marriages before and didn't have the stomach to endure it again. The truth was that we weren't incompatible, merely at the end of our ropes. By our fifth anniversary, we had had two babies, endured a miscarriage, and suffered through the deaths of three of our parents. We worked long hours at stressful jobs. We had no Sunday mornings in bed (I worked Sunday), no late nights out (Steve made early rounds). God, how I envied the couples with time for each other. I imagined them in their kitchens making dinner and talking about their day over companionable glasses of wine. Our kitchen was more like a field headquarters as I rushed around on fast forward trying to get us fed before bedtime.

Then neighbors offered to take our kids so we could get away for occasional weekends if we would take their boys for weekends in return. We grabbed the chance with mixed feelings. We needed to get away; I feared that once we did, we would have the irrevocable fight. Each time I deposited the babies and their paraphernalia, I got into the car praying we would still want to be with each other. But we did. Those weekends were the closest we came to the years-before-children that we never had in our headlong rush into parenthood. We rode our bikes down country roads, popping tires and sprawling in fields filled with Queen Anne's lace. We read in bed. We hiked. We talked each other into spending money on clothes we coveted, a sheepskin jacket for Steve, white silk pants for me.

One evening in Door County, in northern Wisconsin, we sat on the rocks along Green Bay as a storm broke over the town of Menominee on the other shore. We were edgy. Steve had hurt his knee trying to jog and I was feeling guilty because I had pushed him to run with me. We silently watched the lightning flash pink against the blue-gray sky. Thunderheads boiled up, black on the bottom, their rolling tops outlined in an eerie putty-pink. Each flash backlit the town against the darkening sky. I took his hand and we sat in silence at the water's edge until the storm drifted away. Those moments together, some as brief and as illuminating as the lightning over Green Bay, sent us home renewed.

Steve understood that our problems grew from our harried circumstances, not our personalities. Eventually they would fade away. Steve may have hated me at times, but he rarely doubted the marriage would hold. I often stared at the phone, wondering whether to call the lawyer. I was afraid that once I said, "I want out," I could never take the words back. While I believed we were hopelessly mismatched, bound by a perverse chemistry, chosen by a Cupid with a rotten sense of humor, Steve saw that we were alike where it counted. My problem, he said, was that I confused personality and character. "Our values are the same," he insisted, "that's what keeps us together."

After we had been married ten years, we bought an old house. We moved in exhausted; we would leave five years later, healed. The children were older, our jobs were under control, and we were able to catch our breath. The house needed lots of repairs and working together gave us enough projects in common to last a lifetime. We caulked side by side. We put up shelves and lugged heavy pieces of furniture from room to room. Steve dug up the bedraggled flower beds and I replanted them. It was comforting to work with him, to see the quiet way he concentrated on a job until it was done. We talked about how we would spend our money if we won the lottery. After work, we went to soccer games and Little League games and watched our children run through the hazy, golden Midwestern twilight. We took great comfort in the healing routine of ordinary tasks. We took pleasure in doing simple things together. We survived.

So what bonds me to Steve? I finally saw how lucky I was to find a man of real substance, one who shares my longings for home and family. The household sustains him. Children thrill him. He sprawls on the couch with them, rubbing their heads and watching the Yankees blow another game. I love that he loves children, that he can spend a morning on the beach looking for rocks with our friend's eight-year-old, both of them humming tunelessly, showing each other pebbles, holding hands as they pick their way across the stony sand. I love that he went through my sister's wedding with her friend's eight-day-old baby draped on his shoulder.

I trust him, which isn't as obvious as it sounds. He can't tell lies, not even to the phone company. He picks up dimes from the sidewalk and looks around to see who dropped them. He has a generous heart. He lends his clothes, the house, cars, money. A draft horse of a man, he is a puller, a prodigious worker, one for the long haul. He doesn't complain. He believes he can do anything. He is calm. I love that.

He is loyal, even when he has misgivings. When I quit my job to free-lance, he thought I was wrong—I wasn't—but he supported me emotionally and financially. That made it easier for me to stop free-lancing and get a steady job when he wanted to go back to school. When he needed to move on, I cried but I moved from Chicago, a city I love. In turn, he took the job near New York because it was better for me, though he really wanted to live in a smaller town.

Little things endear him to me. He says, "I'm sorry." He goes to Japanese restaurants with me. He gets down on all fours and talks to the dog. He ties great knots. His eyes are bright blue. When we have a drink, he still says, "Here's lookin' at you, kid," waits for my face to curdle because I can't stand the expression, and bursts out laughing. He plays tennis in black business socks and doesn't care that he looks funny. He still does somersaults off the diving board and never looks down.

Believe me when I say that I love this man in a way that is richer and deeper than anything I imagined when we got married. We are like the broken bone—bumpy but strong in the healed places. It is our years together that I love, the things he did for me, the times I rose to the occasion. I love that we lie together whispering before we fall asleep, the familiarity of his body next to mine. I love that he will rub my head for a half hour and not ask me to rub him back.

Am I saying we are a pair of old farts? That we have

traded in passion for coziness? That we have settled for less? No. What we have is not ordinary, not trivial at all, though it took me a long time to respect the old couple on the dock. Like them, we were lucky to find love and comfort in the day-to-day life we make for ourselves. Looking for quicksilver, we seem to have found bedrock. Our lives have converged.

The Authors

Laurie Abraham, twenty-eight, is a former reporter for the *Chicago Reporter*, where she wrote about issues related to race, poverty, and health. She was the youngest writer in *Reinventing Home*, a collection of essays about domestic life published in 1990, and is the author of a book on health care access for four generations of a poor urban family published by the University of Chicago in 1993. She is presently at Yale Law School as recipient of a fellowship for journalists. "This book is a celebration of women's purposeful, pragmatic, and ultimately transcendent approach to love. One writer, a male it so happens, expressed that in a way that inspired me as I wrote these essays. Women recognize, he said, that 'love does not stop being love because it is a power struggle or because it is full of inglorious defeat. The real militarists of love are women.'"

Laura Green, fifty, has spent over twenty years writing about women and social change for both magazines and newspapers. Currently a hospital publicist, she is a co-editor of and contributor to *Reinventing Home*. After leaving daily journalism, she was senior editor of *Chicago Magazine*, and an assistant professor at Northwestern University's Medill School of Journalism.

She lives near New York with her husband and teenage son, and has a daughter in college. "When you sit down to write an essay it gives you the opportunity and the obligation to look at things in a fresh light. When you do that, you can live a little more widely. It's part of the process of reinventing ourselves."

Magda Krance, thirty-seven, is married and the mother of a toddler-age son. A freelance writer for twelve years, she works in public relations for Lyric Opera of Chicago. She is the author of the classic tell-all profile of syndicated columnist and author Bob Greene published in *Spy* magazine, and also has written for *Time* magazine, the *New York Times*, *The Washington Post*, Chicago newspapers, *Self*, *People*, and other national publications. She has sung professionally for several years, most recently with His Majestie's Clerkes and Basically Bach. When she was invited to work on this book she was in the final stages of pregnancy, and says, "The last thing on my mind was writing about love, lust, sex, or romance, but that all changed. Once I started thinking and writing on the subjects, I couldn't stop—when I could find time between diaper changes and feedings to get to my word processor, that is."

Janice Rosenberg, forty-five, married at twenty-three and is still married to the same husband, whom she met in college. Janice says it took her decades to unlearn others' opinions of her and to form new ones she could live with. She says she represents the traditional woman who has had to change. She works as a freelance writer specializing in health subjects and is a contributor to *Reinventing Home*. She has two sons in college. "Writing this book was like being part of a jazz ensemble. One musician would play and another person would take off from there and build on a new image that incorporated the old. In the end, what we wrote had elements of our own experiences and others' lives. No one dominated and we really learned from each other."

Janice Somerville, thirty-one, is a travel addict whose reporting jobs have taken her to the finest restaurants in Paris and to refugee camps in Malawi. She now works for *American Medical News*. She is thankful she passed through her twenties without the pressure to marry. While many of her friends may be commitment shy because of their parents' traumatic divorces, she wonders if she is overly cautious because her parents have had such a great marriage. She confesses that at a recent wedding, instead of hiding in the back when the bouquet was thrown, she lunged through the crowd to grab it. "Whether you think with your head, your heart, or some other part of your anatomy (or ideally all three), isn't nearly as important as knowing the difference. Then it's far easier to make the right choices."

Carroll Stoner, forty-nine, had a twenty-year career in newspapers and was an assistant managing editor of the *Chicago Sun-Times*, where she won the Penney-Missouri Award as editor of the nation's best feature section. She is the co-author of *All God's Children*, about religious cults in America, and author of *Weddings for Grownups* (Chronicle, 1993), about weddings as meaningful ceremonies and celebrations. She writes about subjects related to roots and community and family, and originated the ideas for *Reinventing Home* and *Reinventing Love*. A Minnesotan now living in Chicago, she has been married, for the second time, for over twenty years, and is the mother of a grown son and a pre-teenage daughter. "The important thing for women now is to tell the absolute truth—especially to ourselves—about love and sex and all their permutations. Only then can we lay claim to our own lives."

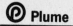

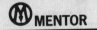 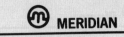